Patient Counseling Handbook

A Comprehensive Guide to Empowering Patients Through Education and Support

www.lulu.com
Lulu Press, Inc
627 Davis Drive, Suite 300,
Morrisville, NC 27560.

Author Affiliations

Ms. Aaska Patel,
Department of Pharmacy Practice,
Anand Pharmacy College,
Anand, Gujarat, India – 388001.

Ms. Trusha Prajapati,
Department of Pharmacy Practice,
Anand Pharmacy College,
Anand, Gujarat, India – 388001.

Mr. Pranshu Pareek,
Department of Pharmacy Practice,
Anand Pharmacy College,
Anand, Gujarat, India – 388001.

Ms. Yagni Master,
Department of Pharmacy Practice,
Anand Pharmacy College,
Anand, Gujarat, India – 388001.

First Printing: 2023

ISBN: 978-1-312-22635-7

Copyright License @ Aaska Patel

This book has been published with all reasonable efforts to make the material error-free after the author's consent. No part of this book shall be used or reproduced in any manner, without the author's permission, except for brief quotations embodied in critical articles and reviews.

The Author of this book is solely responsible and liable for its content, including but not limited to the views, representations, descriptions, statements, information, opinions, and references ["Content"]. The Content of this book shall not constitute or be construed or deemed to reflect the opinion or expression of the Publisher or Editor. Neither the Publisher nor Editor endorse or approve the Content of this book or guarantee the reliability, accuracy, or completeness of the Content published herein and do not make any representations or warranties of any kind, express or implied, including but not limited to the implied warranties of merchantability, fitness for a particular purpose. The Publisher and Editor shall not be liable whatsoever for any errors or omissions, whether such errors or omissions result from negligence, accident, or any other cause or claims for loss or damages of any kind, including without limitation, indirect or consequential loss or damage arising out of use, inability to use, or about the reliability, accuracy or sufficiency of the information contained in this book. This book was written based on Intelligence with the support of various sources.

Patient Counseling Handbook:

A Comprehensive Guide to Empowering Patients Through Education and Support

By

Ms. Aaska Patel,

Ms. Trusha Prajapati,

Mr. Pranshu Pareek,

Ms. Yagni Master.

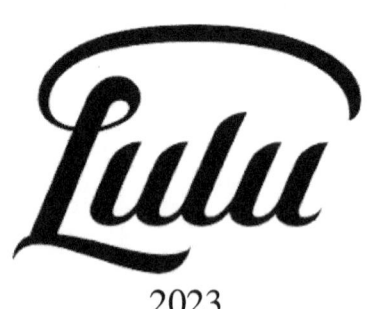

2023

About the Author

Ms. Aaska Rakeshkumar Patel (Pharm. D) authored a few topics for the book "Drug Interaction." She was certified and trained in ICH GCP E6 Guidelines, NDCT Rules 2019, and ICMR Guidelines 2017 and did the certification course on the pharmacovigilance program in 2021. She also attended and presented at national conferences.

Ms. Trusha S. Prajapati (Pharm. D) authored two books and published one case report in a national journal. She is certified and trained in ICH GCP E6 Guidelines, NDCT Rules 2019, and ICMR Guidelines 2017. She also attended a national conference and did the certification course on the pharmacovigilance program.

Mr. Pranshu Pareek (Pharm. D) authored a few topics for the book "Drug-interaction." He was certified and trained in ICH GCP E6 Guidelines, NDCT Rules 2019, and ICMR Guidelines 2017 and did the certification course on the pharmacovigilance program. He also completed some studies at a pharma state academy. She also attended and presented at national conferences.

Ms. Yagni H Master (Pharm. D) authored a few topics for the book "Drug Interaction." She also published one case report in a national journal. She was certified and trained in ICH GCP E6 Guidelines, NDCT Rules 2019, and ICMR Guidelines 2017 and did the certification course on the pharmacovigilance program. She also attended and presented at national conferences.

About Book

In a world where health and wellness are paramount, effective patient counseling promotes informed decision-making and a proactive approach toward well-being. The "Patient Counseling Handbook: A Comprehensive Guide to Empowering Patients Through Education and Support" is a definitive resource designed to equip healthcare professionals and caregivers with the tools to engage, educate, and empower patients on their journey to better health.

Table of Contents

1. Introduction to Patient Counseling 1
    1.1 The Importance of Patient Education 1
        1.1.1 Benefits of Patient Education: 1
        1.1.2. Role of Healthcare Providers in Patient Education 2
    1.2 Effective Communication Techniques 3
        1.2.1 Importance of Effective Communication in Patient Counseling . 3
        1.2.2 Techniques for Effective Communication in Patient Counseling. 4
    1.3 Building Trust and Rapport 5
        1.3.1 Importance of Building Trust and Rapport 5
        1.3.2 Strategies for Building Trust and Rapport 6
2. Understanding Medical Conditions 8
    2.1 Common Medical Terminology 8
        2.1.1 Importance of Common Medical Terminology 8
        2.1.2 Common Components of Medical Terminology 9
        2.1.3 Examples of Common Medical Terminology 9
    2.2 Overview of Major Health Conditions 10
        2.2.1 Cardiovascular Diseases 10
        2.2.2 Respiratory Disorders 12
        2.2.3 Diabetes and Endocrine Disorders 14
        2.2.4 Musculoskeletal Conditions 16
        2.2.5 Neurological Disorders 18
        2.2.6 Gastrointestinal Issues 20
3. Medications and Treatments 22
    3.1 Medication Safety and Compliance 22

- 3.1.1 Medication Safety 22
- 3.1.2 Medication Compliance 23
- 3.2 Dosage Administration 23
  - 3.2.1 Key Principles of Dosage Administration 24
  - 3.2.2 Dosage Forms 24
  - 3.2.3 Dosage Adjustments and Safety 25
- 3.3 Potential Side Effects and Interactions 26
  - 3.3.1 Potential Side Effects 26
  - 3.3.2 Medication Interactions 26
  - 3.3.3 Reducing Risks and Addressing Concerns 27
- 3.4 Non-Pharmacological Treatments 28
  - 3.4.1 Lifestyle Modifications 28
  - 3.4.2 Therapies and Interventions 29
  - 3.4.3 Complementary and Alternative Medicine (CAM) 30
  - 3.4.4 Patient Education and Self-Management 30
- 3.5 Surgical Procedures and Aftercare 31
  - 3.5.1 Surgical Procedures 31
  - 3.5.2 Post-Operative Care and Aftercare 32
- 4. Lifestyle and Wellness 34
  - 4.1 Nutrition and Diet Management 34
    - 4.1.1 Key Principles of Nutrition 34
    - 4.1.2 Dietary Considerations for Specific Conditions 34
    - 4.1.3 Tips for Healthy Eating 35
  - 4.2 Physical Activity and Exercise Guidelines 36
    - 4.2.1 Importance of Physical Activity 36
    - 4.2.2 Physical Activity Guidelines 37

- 4.2.3 Exercise Considerations ... 37
- 4.2.4 Staying Motivated ... 37
- 4.3 Stress Management and Mental Health ... 38
  - 4.3.1 Understanding Stress ... 38
  - 4.3.2 Stress Management Strategies ... 39
  - 4.3.3 Mental Health and Well-Being ... 39
  - 4.3.4 Seeking Help ... 40
- 4.4 Sleep Hygiene and Restful Practices ... 40
  - 4.4.1 Importance of Sleep ... 40
  - 4.4.2 Sleep Hygiene Practices ... 41
  - 4.4.3 Restful Practices ... 42
  - 4.4.4 Seeking Help for Sleep Issues ... 42
- 4.5 Substance Abuse Prevention and Cessation ... 43
  - 4.5.1 Substance Abuse Prevention ... 43
  - 4.5.2 Substance Cessation ... 43
  - 4.5.3 Alcohol and Tobacco Cessation ... 44
  - 4.5.4 Prescription Medication Safety ... 44
  - 4.5.5 Illicit Drugs ... 44
- 5. Special Patient Groups ... 46
  - 5.1 Pediatrics and Childcare ... 46
    - 5.1.1 Well-Baby and Well-Child Visits ... 46
    - 5.1.2 Common Pediatric Health Concerns ... 46
    - 5.1.3 Parenting and Childcare ... 47
    - 5.1.4 Adolescents and Teenagers ... 47
  - 5.2 Geriatrics and Aging Healthfully ... 48
    - 5.2.1 Health Considerations in Geriatrics ... 48

- 5.2.2 Comprehensive Geriatric Assessment 49
- 5.2.3 Age-Related Health Promotion 49
- 5.2.4 Palliative and Hospice Care 49
- 5.2.5 Mental and Emotional Health 50
- 5.3 Pregnancy, Prenatal Care, and Postpartum Support 50
  - 5.3.1 Pregnancy and Prenatal Care 50
  - 5.3.2 Labor and Childbirth 51
  - 5.3.3 Postpartum Support 51
  - 5.3.4 Family Planning and Contraception 52
  - 5.3.5 Preparing for Another Pregnancy 52
  - 5.3.6 Genetic Counseling 52
- 5.4 Chronic Disease Management 52
  - 5.4.1 Understanding Chronic Diseases 53
  - 5.4.2 Chronic Disease Management Strategies 53
  - 5.4.3 Diabetes Management 54
  - 5.4.4 Cardiovascular Disease Management 54
  - 5.4.5 COPD Management 54
- 6. Preventive Care and Screenings 56
  - 6.1 Immunizations and Vaccination Schedules 56
    - 6.1.1 Importance of Immunizations 56
    - 6.1.2 Vaccination Schedules 56
    - 6.1.3 Vaccine Safety 57
    - 6.1.4 Special Considerations 57
  - 6.2 Cancer Screenings and Early Detection 58
    - 6.2.1 Importance of Cancer Screenings 58
    - 6.2.2 Common Cancer Screenings 59

- 6.2.3 Early Detection and Self-Exams ... 59
- 6.2.4 Screening Guidelines ... 59
- 6.2.5 Follow-Up and Treatment ... 60
- 6.3 Routine Health Check-ups and Monitoring ... 60
  - 6.3.1 Importance of Routine Check-ups ... 61
  - 6.3.2 Components of Routine Check-ups ... 61
  - 6.3.3 Monitoring Chronic Conditions ... 62
  - 6.3.4 Age-Related Considerations ... 62
  - 6.3.5 Follow-Up and Communication ... 62
- 7. Health Resources and Support ... 64
  - 7.1 Accessing Healthcare Services ... 64
    - 7.1.1 Primary Care Providers ... 64
    - 7.1.2 Specialists ... 64
    - 7.1.3 Urgent Care and Emergency Services ... 64
    - 7.1.4 Telehealth Services ... 65
    - 7.1.5 Health Insurance ... 65
    - 7.1.6 Community Health Centers ... 65
    - 7.1.7 Prescription Medications ... 65
    - 7.1.8 Patient Portals and Apps ... 66
    - 7.1.9 Health Education and Support ... 66
  - 7.2 Health Insurance and Financial Assistance ... 66
    - 7.2.1 Health Insurance Options ... 66
    - 7.2.2 Understanding Health Insurance ... 67
    - 7.2.3 Financial Assistance and Support ... 67
    - 7.2.4 Applying for Financial Assistance ... 68
    - 7.2.5 Managing Costs ... 68

7.3 Patient Advocacy and Support Groups 69
    7.3.1 Patient Advocacy 69
    7.3.2 Support Groups 70
    7.3.3 Types of Support Groups 70
    7.3.4 How to Access Patient Advocacy and Support 70
    7.3.5 Participation and Benefits 71

7.4 Online Health Information: Reliability and Safety 71
    7.4.1 Importance of Reliable Information 72
    7.4.2 Evaluating Online Health Information 72
    7.4.3 Red Flags for Unreliable Information 72
    7.4.4 Verifying Medical Information 73
    7.4.5 Online Health Communities 73
    7.4.6 Official Health Websites 73
    7.4.7 Telehealth and Virtual Visits 73
    7.4.8 Health Literacy 73

8. Emergency Preparedness and First Aid 75
  8.1 Basic First Aid Techniques 75
    8.1.1 Assessing the Situation 75
    8.1.2 CPR (Cardiopulmonary Resuscitation) 75
    8.1.3 Choking 75
    8.1.4 Bleeding and Wound Care 76
    8.1.5 Burns 76
    8.1.6 Fractures and Sprains 76
    8.1.7 Seizures 76
    8.1.8 Allergic Reactions 77
    8.1.9 Bites and Stings 77

8.2 Creating a Personal Emergency Plan 77
8.2.1 Assess Potential Risks 77
8.2.2 Develop Your Plan 78
8.2.3 Practice and Review 79
8.2.4 Stay Informed 79
8.2.5 Tailor Your Plan 79
8.3 Recognizing Signs of Medical Emergencies 80
8.3.1 Heart Attack 80
8.3.2 Stroke 80
8.3.3 Severe Allergic Reaction (Anaphylaxis) 80
8.3.4 Choking 81
8.3.5 Unconsciousness or Fainting 81
8.3.6 Seizures 81
8.3.7 Difficulty Breathing 81
8.3.8 Bleeding 81
8.3.9 Poisoning 82

9. Appendix 83
9.1 Case Studies 83
9.2 Real-Life Patient Scenarios and Counseling Approaches 84
9.3 Brief on Different types of Patient Counselling Forms 87
9.4 Glossary of Medical Terms 89

References 94

1. Introduction to Patient Counseling

1.1 The Importance of Patient Education

Patient education is a critical component of healthcare that plays a vital role in promoting wellness, preventing illness, and improving overall patient outcomes. It involves providing patients with the necessary information, resources, and guidance to understand their health conditions, make informed decisions about their care, and actively participate in managing their health.

1.1.1 Benefits of Patient Education:

Patient education offers several significant benefits that contribute to the well-being of individuals and the healthcare system as a whole:

- Educated patients are better equipped to take control of their health. When patients clearly understand their conditions, treatment options, and self-care strategies, they are more likely to actively participate in their care, leading to better health outcomes.
- Patients who comprehend the rationale behind their treatment plans and the importance of following medical advice are more likely to adhere to prescribed medications, lifestyle modifications, and follow-up appointments. This adherence enhances the effectiveness of treatment and reduces the risk of complications.
- Informed patients can actively participate in shared decision-making with their healthcare providers. This collaboration allows patients to choose treatment options that align with their values, preferences, and goals, leading to more personalized and effective care.
- Patient education is a powerful tool for preventing the onset or progression of certain diseases. By promoting healthy behaviors, proper nutrition, regular exercise, and early detection, patient

- education can help individuals reduce their risk of chronic conditions.
- When patients are knowledgeable about their conditions and treatment plans, they are less likely to require hospitalization or emergency care due to preventable complications. This can lead to cost savings for both patients and the healthcare system.
- Educated patients are better equipped to manage symptoms, cope with the challenges of chronic illness, and maintain a higher quality of life. They are more likely to experience reduced anxiety and increased confidence in managing their health.
- Understanding medication instructions, potential side effects, and proper use of medical devices contributes to patient safety. Education helps prevent medication errors and promotes safe self-administration of treatments.
- Patient education builds knowledge and skills beyond immediate medical concerns. It equips patients with the tools they need to make informed decisions about their health throughout their lives.

1.1.2. Role of Healthcare Providers in Patient Education

Healthcare providers, including doctors, nurses, pharmacists, and other healthcare team members, are crucial in patient education. They should communicate information, tailor instruction to the patient's level of understanding, and encourage patients to ask questions. Effective patient education involves:

- Understanding the patient's current knowledge, beliefs, and learning readiness.
- Explaining medical concepts in simple language, using visual aids if necessary.
- Tailoring Education to the patient's cultural background, literacy level, and personal preferences.
- Providing information at multiple points of care and reinforcing critical points during follow-up visits.
- Involving patients in decision-making and goal setting.

- Offering written materials, online resources, and reliable sources of information.
- Assessing the patient's comprehension and addressing any misconceptions.

Patient education is a cornerstone of effective healthcare delivery. By empowering patients with knowledge and skills, healthcare providers contribute to improved health outcomes, increased patient satisfaction, and a more efficient healthcare system.

1.2 Effective Communication Techniques

Effective communication is a fundamental skill in patient counseling that allows healthcare providers to establish trust, facilitate understanding, and promote positive patient outcomes. Communicating empathetically and respectfully is essential for building strong patient-provider relationships and ensuring patients are actively engaged in their healthcare journey.

1.2.1 Importance of Effective Communication in Patient Counseling

Effective communication in patient counseling serves several critical purposes.

- Clear and empathetic communication helps build trust between patients and healthcare providers. Patients who feel understood and valued are likelier to share important information and actively participate in their care.
- Complex medical information can be overwhelming for patients. Effective communication techniques make this information understandable, ensuring patients comprehend their conditions, treatment options, and care plans.
- Patients are more likely to follow treatment plans and make necessary lifestyle changes when they understand the rationale

behind the recommendations. Effective communication can motivate patients to adhere to prescribed therapies and behaviors.
- Informed patients are better equipped to make decisions that align with their values and preferences. Effective communication allows patients to engage in shared decision-making with their healthcare providers actively.
- Patients may have questions, fears, or doubts about their health. Effective communication provides a platform for patients to voice their concerns, enabling providers to address them and alleviate anxiety.
- Patients who receive clear instructions and guidance on self-care are more likely to manage their conditions effectively and prevent complications.

1.2.2 Techniques for Effective Communication in Patient Counseling

- Pay close attention to the patient, make eye contact, and provide verbal and nonverbal cues to show you are engaged and listening. Avoid interrupting and allow the patient to express their thoughts and concerns thoroughly.
- Demonstrate genuine empathy for the patient's emotions and concerns. Use supportive language, acknowledge their feelings, and treat them respectfully and respectfully.
- Explain medical concepts and treatment plans using simple, jargon-free language. Analogies and metaphors can help patients relate to unfamiliar information.
- Ask questions encouraging patients to provide detailed responses, allowing you to gather comprehensive information and understand their perspectives.
- Summarize the discussion's main points to ensure you and the patient understand the information shared. This also provides an opportunity to address any misconceptions.

- ❖ Pay attention to your tone of voice, facial expressions, and body language. These cues can convey empathy, reassurance, and attentiveness.
- ❖ Visual aids such as diagrams, models, or written materials can help reinforce explanations and make complex information more accessible.
- ❖ Encourage patients to ask questions and provide feedback on their understanding. This allows you to gauge their comprehension and address any gaps in knowledge.
- ❖ Be mindful of the patient's cultural background and preferences. Adapt your communication style to accommodate cultural norms and beliefs.
- ❖ Allocate sufficient time for counseling sessions to avoid rushing through important information. Patients should feel that their concerns are being heard and addressed.

Effective communication techniques are essential for successful patient counseling. By using active listening, empathy, plain language, and other strategies, healthcare providers can establish strong relationships, improve patient understanding, and facilitate informed decision-making.

1.3 Building Trust and Rapport

Building trust and rapport is a cornerstone of effective patient counseling. Establishing a trusting relationship between healthcare providers and patients forms the foundation for open communication, collaboration, and successful healthcare outcomes.

1.3.1 Importance of Building Trust and Rapport

- ➢ Trust and rapport create an environment where patients feel comfortable sharing their concerns, symptoms, and personal information. This open communication allows healthcare providers to gather accurate and comprehensive information for diagnosis and treatment.

- When patients trust their healthcare providers, they are more likely to actively participate in their care plans, follow medical advice, and make informed decisions about their health.
- A trusting relationship enhances patient adherence to prescribed treatments, medications, and lifestyle modifications. Patients are more likely to follow recommendations when they believe in the provider's expertise and intentions.
- Patients are more receptive to counseling and Education when a strong rapport is established. This facilitates the exchange of information and increases the likelihood of patients understanding and applying the guidance provided.
- Trust and rapport allow healthcare providers to address patients' emotional and psychological needs. Patients who feel understood and supported can better cope with the challenges of illness.
- A trusting relationship enables shared decision-making between patients and providers. Patients are more likely to discuss treatment options, risks, and benefits when they trust their provider has their best interests at heart.

1.3.2 Strategies for Building Trust and Rapport

- Please observe the patient, demonstrate empathy, and validate their feelings. Show that you are genuinely interested in understanding their concerns.
- Treat every patient respectfully, regardless of background, beliefs, or health condition. Maintain a nonjudgmental attitude and use polite language.
- Consistently deliver accurate information, follow promises, and provide reliable care. Patients value consistency and reliability in their healthcare interactions.
- Put yourself in the patient's shoes, acknowledge their emotions, and show understanding of their experiences. Empathy helps build a solid emotional connection.

- ➢ Be open and honest about treatment options, potential risks, and uncertainties. Transparency fosters trust by demonstrating that you have the patient's best interests in mind.
- ➢ Respect the patient's autonomy and involve them in decision-making. Provide information to empower them to make choices about their care.
- ➢ Allocate sufficient time for patient interactions, and be available to address questions or concerns. Patients appreciate feeling heard and valued.
- ➢ Respect patient privacy and maintain strict confidentiality. Patients must trust that their personal and medical information will be kept confidential.
- ➢ Be sensitive to cultural differences and tailor your communication and care approach to meet patients' cultural needs and preferences.
- ➢ Address patients by their preferred names and take an interest in their personal lives beyond their medical conditions. This humanizes the interaction and builds rapport.
- ➢ Involve patients in decisions about their care, explain the rationale behind recommendations, and ensure they understand and agree with the proposed plans.

Building trust and rapport is essential for effective patient counseling. By demonstrating empathy, respect, transparency, and cultural competence, healthcare providers can create a positive and supportive environment that promotes open communication, informed decision-making, and successful healthcare outcomes.

2. Understanding Medical Conditions

2.1 Common Medical Terminology

Understanding medical terminology is crucial for healthcare providers and patients to communicate effectively about medical conditions, diagnoses, treatments, and procedures. Medical terminology consists of specialized words and phrases that convey precise meanings and facilitate accurate and efficient communication within the healthcare field.

2.1.1 Importance of Common Medical Terminology

Medical terminology provides a standardized and precise way to describe complex medical concepts. Using specific terms reduces ambiguity and ensures that healthcare professionals and patients understand each other clearly.

Medical terminology is essential for accurate and consistent documentation of patient information, diagnoses, treatments, and outcomes. This contributes to comprehensive and organized medical records.

Medical terminology enables healthcare providers to communicate efficiently and accurately with each other. It also allows patients to comprehend their conditions and treatment plans, fostering better patient-provider interactions.

Proficiency in medical terminology enhances the credibility and professionalism of healthcare providers. It demonstrates a level of expertise and competence within the field.

Medical students, trainees, and patients can use medical terminology to access reliable medical resources, research, and educational materials. It facilitates understanding and engagement in the learning process.

2.1.2 Common Components of Medical Terminology

Root Words (Roots): These are the core words that provide the fundamental meaning of a medical term. For example, "cardi-" is the root of terms related to the heart.

Prefixes: Prefixes are added to the beginning of a root word to modify its meaning. For instance, "hyper-" is a prefix that means excessive, as in "hypertension" (high blood pressure).

Suffixes: Suffixes are added to the end of a root word to modify its meaning or indicate a condition, procedure, or part of the body. For example, "itis" is a suffix that implies inflammation, as in "gastritis" (inflammation of the stomach).

Combining Vowels: Vowels are used to make the pronunciation of medical terms easier and to connect word parts. For example, "cardi/o" combines the root "cardi-" with the vowel "-o" to form the term for the heart.

2.1.3 Examples of Common Medical Terminology

Gastroenteritis: "Gastro-" (related to the stomach) + "enter-" (related to the intestines) + "-itis" (inflammation). Refers to inflammation of the stomach and intestines.

Hemoglobin: "Hemo-" (related to blood) + "globin" (a protein component). Refers to the protein in red blood cells that carries oxygen.

Dermatology: "Derm-" (related to the skin) + "-ology" (the study of). Refers to the medical specialty focused on skin conditions.

Hypothyroidism: "Hypo-" (below normal) + "thyroid" (a gland in the neck) + "-ism" (condition). Refers to an underactive thyroid gland.

Osteoporosis: "Osteo-" (related to bone) + "-porosis" (porous condition). Refers to a condition of weakened and brittle bones.

Cardiovascular: "Cardio-" (related to the heart) + "vascular" (related to blood vessels). Refers to the system involving the heart and blood vessels.

Learning and using standard medical terminology helps healthcare professionals and patients communicate effectively, ensuring accurate and comprehensive discussions about medical conditions and treatments. It is a valuable skill that supports quality healthcare delivery and promotes patient understanding.

2.2 Overview of Major Health Conditions

An overview of significant health conditions encompasses various diseases and disorders that affect individuals' well-being and require medical attention. Here is a brief overview of some common primary health conditions across various categories:

2.2.1 Cardiovascular Diseases

Cardiovascular diseases (CVD) are a group of disorders that affect the heart and blood vessels. They are among the leading causes of death and disability worldwide. Cardiovascular diseases encompass a range of conditions that can significantly impact an individual's health and well-being. Here is an overview of some common cardiovascular diseases:

Coronary Artery Disease (CAD): CAD occurs when the blood vessels that supply the heart (coronary arteries) become narrowed or blocked due to plaque buildup. This can lead to angina (chest pain) or a heart attack (myocardial infarction) if the blood flow is restricted.

Hypertension (High Blood Pressure): Hypertension is a condition where the force of blood against the artery walls is consistently too high. It can strain the heart, damage blood vessels, and increase the risk of heart disease, stroke, and other complications.

Heart Failure: Heart failure occurs when the heart cannot pump blood effectively, leading to fatigue, shortness of breath, fluid retention, and swelling.

Arrhythmias: Arrhythmias are abnormal heart rhythms. They can manifest as a slow heartbeat (bradycardia), a fast heartbeat (tachycardia), or irregular heartbeats (atrial fibrillation, ventricular fibrillation).

Valvular Heart Diseases: These conditions involve damage or dysfunction of the heart valves, affecting blood flow within the heart. Examples include aortic stenosis and mitral regurgitation.

Peripheral Artery Disease (PAD): PAD occurs when there is reduced blood flow to the extremities (usually the legs) due to narrowed or blocked arteries. It can cause leg pain, slow wound healing, and increase the risk of amputation.

Stroke: A stroke occurs when the blood supply to the brain is disrupted, leading to brain damage. Ischemic strokes result from blocked blood vessels, while hemorrhagic strokes involve bleeding within the brain.

Congenital Heart Defects: These structural abnormalities at birth affect the heart's structure and function. They can range from mild to severe and may require surgical intervention.

Prevention and management of cardiovascular diseases involve lifestyle modifications (such as a healthy diet, regular exercise, and smoking cessation), medications, medical procedures (e.g., angioplasty, bypass surgery), and ongoing medical supervision.

Early detection and timely intervention are crucial in reducing the impact of cardiovascular diseases and improving outcomes.

Healthcare providers are pivotal in educating patients about cardiovascular health, assessing risk factors, and developing personalized treatment plans to effectively address and manage these conditions.

2.2.2 Respiratory Disorders

Respiratory disorders encompass a variety of conditions that affect the lungs and the respiratory system. These disorders can significantly impact an individual's ability to breathe, ranging from mild to severe. Here is an overview of some common respiratory disorders:

Asthma: Asthma is a chronic inflammatory disease of the airways that leads to recurrent episodes of wheezing, coughing, shortness of breath, and chest tightness. Allergens, exercise, cold air, or respiratory infections can trigger these symptoms.

Chronic Obstructive Pulmonary Disease (COPD): COPD is a progressive lung disease that includes chronic bronchitis and emphysema. It is characterized by persistent airflow limitation, leading to symptoms like cough, sputum production, and shortness of breath.

Chronic Bronchitis: This type of COPD is characterized by chronic inflammation of the bronchial tubes, leading to increased mucus production and cough that persists for most days of the month for at least three months in two consecutive years.

Emphysema: Emphysema is another type of COPD where the air sacs (alveoli) in the lungs become damaged, leading to reduced lung elasticity and impaired gas exchange.

Pneumonia: Pneumonia is an infection that causes inflammation in the lungs' air sacs. It can be caused by bacteria, viruses, fungi, or other microorganisms, leading to symptoms like fever, cough, chest pain, and difficulty breathing.

Interstitial Lung Disease: This group of disorders involves inflammation and scarring of the lung tissue (interstitium), affecting the lungs' ability to expand and contract properly.

Lung Cancer: Lung cancer is a malignant tumor that originates in the lungs and can spread to other body parts. It is often linked to smoking but can also occur in non-smokers.

Pulmonary Hypertension: Pulmonary hypertension is high blood pressure in the lungs' arteries, which strains the heart and can lead to heart failure.

Obstructive Sleep Apnea: Sleep apnea is characterized by pauses in breathing during sleep due to a blocked or narrowed airway. It leads to disrupted sleep and daytime fatigue.

Cystic Fibrosis: Cystic fibrosis is a genetic disorder that affects the lungs and digestive system. It leads to thick, sticky mucus production, which can obstruct airways and cause respiratory infections.

Acute Respiratory Distress Syndrome (ARDS): ARDS is a severe lung condition characterized by rapid fluid accumulation, leading to severe difficulty breathing and low oxygen levels.

Management of respiratory disorders may involve lifestyle modifications, medications (such as bronchodilators, anti-inflammatory drugs, and antibiotics), oxygen therapy, pulmonary rehabilitation, and, in some cases, surgical interventions. Early diagnosis and appropriate management are essential to improve the quality of life and outcomes for individuals with respiratory disorders.

Healthcare providers are crucial in diagnosing, treating, and educating patients about these conditions.

2.2.3 Diabetes and Endocrine Disorders

Diabetes and endocrine disorders involve disruptions in the body's hormonal balance, which can lead to various health issues. Hormones are crucial in regulating various bodily functions, and imbalances can significantly affect metabolism, growth, development, and overall health. Here is an overview of Diabetes and some common endocrine disorders:

Diabetes

Diabetes is a group of chronic metabolic disorders characterized by high blood sugar levels (hyperglycemia) due to either insufficient insulin production or ineffective use by the body. There are three main types of Diabetes:

Type 1 Diabetes: An autoimmune condition where the immune system attacks and destroys the insulin-producing cells in the pancreas. People with type 1 diabetes require insulin injections or an insulin pump to manage their blood sugar levels.

Type 2 Diabetes: This is the most common type of Diabetes, often associated with lifestyle factors such as obesity and sedentary behavior. In type 2 diabetes, the body becomes resistant to the effects of insulin, and the pancreas may not produce enough insulin to compensate.

Gestational Diabetes: Occurs during pregnancy and is characterized by elevated blood sugar levels. It usually resolves after childbirth but increases the risk of developing type 2 diabetes later in life.

Other Endocrine Disorders

Hypothyroidism: A condition where the thyroid gland does not produce enough thyroid hormone, leading to symptoms such as fatigue, weight gain, and cold sensitivity.

Hyperthyroidism: The thyroid gland produces excessive amounts of thyroid hormone, leading to symptoms like weight loss, rapid heartbeat, and heat intolerance.

Cushing's Syndrome: Caused by prolonged exposure to high levels of the hormone cortisol, resulting in symptoms like weight gain, facial rounding, and skin thinning.

Addison's Disease: Occurs when the adrenal glands do not produce enough cortisol and sometimes aldosterone. Symptoms include fatigue, weight loss, and low blood pressure.

Polycystic Ovary Syndrome (PCOS): A hormonal disorder common in women of reproductive age, characterized by irregular periods, excess hair growth, acne, and polycystic ovaries.

Hyperparathyroidism: The parathyroid glands produce too much parathyroid hormone, leading to high levels of calcium in the blood and potential bone and kidney issues.

Hypopituitarism: Reduced function of the pituitary gland, affecting the production of various hormones that regulate growth, metabolism, and reproduction.

Diabetes Insipidus: A condition where the kidneys cannot properly conserve water, leading to excessive thirst and urination.

Thyroid Nodules and Cancer: Abnormal growths in the thyroid gland, which can be benign nodules or, in some cases, cancerous tumors.

Management of diabetes and endocrine disorders involves a combination of medication, lifestyle modifications, hormone replacement therapy, and regular medical monitoring. Early diagnosis and effective leadership are crucial for minimizing complications and improving the quality of life for individuals with these conditions. Healthcare providers play a central role in diagnosing, treating, and educating patients about Diabetes and endocrine disorders.

2.2.4 Musculoskeletal Conditions

Musculoskeletal conditions refer to a group of disorders that affect the body's bones, muscles, joints, and connective tissues. These conditions can cause pain, discomfort, limited mobility, and other symptoms that impact an individual's ability to perform daily activities. Here is an overview of some common musculoskeletal conditions:

Osteoarthritis (OA): Osteoarthritis is a degenerative joint disease that occurs when the protective cartilage cushions the ends of bones and wears down over time. It can lead to joint pain, stiffness, and reduced range of motion, often affecting weight-bearing joints such as the knees, hips, and spine.

Rheumatoid Arthritis (RA): Rheumatoid arthritis is an autoimmune disorder where the immune system mistakenly attacks the synovium (the lining of the membranes surrounding joints), causing inflammation, pain, swelling, and joint deformities.

Osteoporosis: Osteoporosis is characterized by weakened bones, decreased bone density, and increased risk of fractures. It is more common in older adults, particularly postmenopausal women, and can lead to fractures even from minor trauma.

Fibromyalgia: Fibromyalgia is a chronic disorder characterized by widespread musculoskeletal pain, fatigue, and tenderness. It often coexists with other conditions, such as depression and anxiety.

Lupus (Systemic Lupus Erythematosus): Lupus is an autoimmune disease affecting multiple systems, including the musculoskeletal system. Joint pain, swelling, and stiffness are common symptoms.

Ankylosing Spondylitis: Ankylosing spondylitis is an inflammatory arthritis that primarily affects the spine, causing pain and stiffness. Over time, it can lead to the fusion of the spine's vertebrae.

Gout: A gout is a form of arthritis characterized by sudden and severe joint pain, often affecting the big toe. It is caused by the buildup of uric acid crystals in the joints.

Carpal Tunnel Syndrome: Carpal tunnel syndrome is when the median nerve in the wrist becomes compressed, leading to numbness, tingling, and weakness in the hand and fingers.

Herniated Disc (Slipped Disc): A herniated disc occurs when the soft inner portion of a spinal disc pushes through the more rigid outer layer, potentially causing back pain and nerve compression.

Scoliosis: Scoliosis is an abnormal curvature of the spine, which can lead to uneven shoulders, hips and potential lung and heart issues if severe.

Management of musculoskeletal conditions may involve a combination of medications (such as pain relievers and anti-inflammatories), physical therapy, exercise, lifestyle modifications, assistive devices, and, in some cases, surgical interventions. Early diagnosis and appropriate management are essential to improve function, reduce pain, and enhance the quality of life for individuals with musculoskeletal conditions. Healthcare providers are crucial in diagnosing, treating, and educating patients about these conditions and their management options.

2.2.5 Neurological Disorders

Neurological disorders encompass various conditions that affect the nervous system, including the brain, spinal cord, and peripheral nerves. These disorders can impact bodily functions like movement, sensation, cognition, and communication. Here is an overview of some common neurological disorders:

Alzheimer's Disease: Alzheimer's is a progressive neurodegenerative disorder affecting memory, thinking, and behavior. It is the most common cause of dementia in older adults.

Parkinson's Disease: Parkinson's disease is a movement disorder characterized by tremors, rigidity, bradykinesia (slowed movement), and postural instability. It results from the loss of dopamine-producing cells in the brain.

Multiple Sclerosis (MS): Multiple sclerosis is an autoimmune disease where the immune system attacks the protective myelin sheath that covers nerve fibers. This can lead to a wide range of symptoms, including fatigue, muscle weakness, and problems with coordination and balance.

Epilepsy: Epilepsy is a neurological disorder characterized by recurrent seizures, abnormal bursts of brain electrical activity.

Migraine: Migraine is a headache characterized by severe, throbbing pain often accompanied by other symptoms like nausea, vomiting, and sensitivity to light and sound.

Amyotrophic Lateral Sclerosis (ALS): ALS, also known as Lou Gehrig's disease, is a progressive neurodegenerative disorder that affects nerve cells in the brain and spinal cord, leading to muscle weakness and paralysis.

Stroke: A stroke occurs when blood flow to the brain is disrupted, leading to brain damage. Ischemic strokes result from blocked blood vessels, while hemorrhagic strokes involve bleeding within the brain.

Neuropathy: Neuropathy is a term used to describe conditions that affect the peripheral nerves, leading to symptoms like numbness, tingling, and weakness in the extremities.

Cerebral Palsy: Cerebral palsy is a group of disorders that affect movement, muscle tone, and posture. It is often caused by brain damage before or during birth.

Huntington's Disease: Huntington's disease is an inherited disorder that leads to the progressive breakdown of nerve cells in the brain, resulting in movement problems, cognitive decline, and behavioral changes.

Tourette Syndrome: Tourette syndrome is a neurological disorder characterized by repetitive, involuntary movements and vocalizations known as tics.

Neurodevelopmental Disorders: These include conditions like autism spectrum disorder, attention-deficit/hyperactivity disorder (ADHD), and intellectual disabilities, which affect brain development and often manifest in childhood.

Neurological disorders can profoundly impact an individual's daily life and functioning. Management may involve a combination of medications, physical therapy, occupational therapy, speech therapy, counseling, and other supportive interventions. Early diagnosis and appropriate management are crucial to improving the quality of life for individuals with neurological disorders. Healthcare providers play a central role in diagnosing, treating, and educating patients and their families about these conditions.

2.2.6 Gastrointestinal Issues

Gastrointestinal (GI) issues refer to a wide range of disorders that affect the digestive system, including the stomach, intestines, liver, gallbladder, and pancreas. These conditions can cause various symptoms related to digestion, nutrient absorption, and waste elimination. Here is an overview of some common gastrointestinal issues:

Gastroesophageal Reflux Disease (GERD): GERD is a chronic condition where stomach acid flows back into the esophagus, causing heartburn, regurgitation, and other symptoms.

Peptic Ulcers: Peptic ulcers are open sores that develop on the inner lining of the stomach, small intestine, or esophagus. They can cause abdominal pain, bloating, and bleeding.

Irritable Bowel Syndrome (IBS): IBS is a functional disorder of the digestive tract characterized by abdominal pain, bloating, and changes in bowel habits such as diarrhea and constipation.

Inflammatory Bowel Disease (IBD): IBD includes Crohn's disease and ulcerative colitis, which are chronic inflammatory conditions that affect the intestines, leading to symptoms like abdominal pain, diarrhea, and weight loss.

Celiac Disease: Celiac disease is an autoimmune disorder where consuming gluten triggers an immune response that damages the small intestine's lining, leading to malabsorption of nutrients.

Gallstones: Gallstones are solid particles that form in the gallbladder, often causing pain, nausea, and other digestive symptoms.

Gastroenteritis: Gastroenteritis is inflammation of the stomach and intestines, usually caused by infection. It leads to symptoms like diarrhea, vomiting, and abdominal cramps.

Hepatitis: Hepatitis is inflammation of the liver, often caused by viral infections (such as hepatitis A, B, or C). It can lead to jaundice, fatigue, and liver damage.

Pancreatitis: Pancreatitis is inflammation of the pancreas, causing abdominal pain, nausea, and vomiting.

Diverticulitis: Diverticulitis is inflammation or infection of small pouches that can form in the colon lining, leading to abdominal pain, fever, and changes in bowel habits.

Gastrointestinal Bleeding: Gastrointestinal bleeding can occur in various parts of the digestive tract and may result in symptoms like black or bloody stools, vomiting blood, and abdominal pain.

Constipation and Diarrhea: These are common digestive symptoms resulting from various underlying causes, such as dietary factors, medications, or underlying medical conditions.

Liver Cirrhosis: Cirrhosis is the scarring of the liver tissue, often caused by chronic liver disease. It can lead to liver dysfunction and complications.

    GI issues can significantly impact an individual's daily life and overall well-being. Management may involve dietary modifications, medications, lifestyle changes, and, in some cases, surgical interventions. Early diagnosis and appropriate management are crucial to prevent complications and improve the quality of life for individuals with gastrointestinal issues. Healthcare providers are central in diagnosing, treating, and educating patients about these conditions and their management options.

3. Medications and Treatments

3.1 Medication Safety and Compliance

Medication safety and compliance are critical aspects of effective healthcare management. Proper use of medications and adherence to prescribed treatment plans are essential for achieving desired health outcomes and preventing potential risks and complications. Here is an overview of medication safety and compliance:

3.1.1 Medication Safety

- ❖ Ensure medications are administered correctly, following the prescribed dosage, route (oral, injection, etc.), and frequency. Use appropriate measuring tools and techniques.
- ❖ Store medications in a cool, dry place, away from direct sunlight and out of the reach of children. Some medicines may require refrigeration.
- ❖ Always read and follow the medication label, including instructions, warnings, and expiration dates. If you have any questions, consult a healthcare provider or pharmacist.
- ❖ Do not self-prescribe or use someone else's medication. Consult a healthcare professional before starting any new medication.
- ❖ Inform your healthcare provider and pharmacist about any allergies or sensitivities you have to medications or their ingredients.
- ❖ Be cautious about potential medication interactions, including prescription, over-the-counter, and herbal supplements. Inform your healthcare provider about all medicines you are taking.
- ❖ Be aware of the potential side effects of medications. If you experience unexpected or severe side effects, contact your healthcare provider.

- Dispose of unused or expired medications correctly to prevent accidental ingestion. Follow local guidelines for safe disposal.

3.1.2 Medication Compliance

- Clearly understand how and when to take your medications. Ask your healthcare provider or pharmacist for clarification if you have any doubts.
- Take medications as prescribed, adhering to the recommended dosage, timing, and duration of treatment.
- Use tools like alarms, pill organizers, or smartphone apps to help you remember to take your medications.
- Discuss any challenges you face with medication administration or potential side effects with your healthcare provider. They may adjust your treatment plan if necessary.
- Understand the purpose of each medication, its potential benefits, and role in managing your condition.
- Ensure you have a sufficient supply of medications and refill prescriptions before running out.
- Collaborate with your healthcare provider in making decisions about your treatment plan. If you have concerns or preferences, discuss them openly.
- Attend follow-up appointments as scheduled to monitor your progress and make any necessary adjustments to your treatment plan.
- Proper medication safety and compliance are crucial for managing health conditions effectively. Engage in open communication with your healthcare provider and pharmacist and actively participate in your healthcare journey to ensure optimal medication use and positive health outcomes.

3.2 Dosage Administration

Dosage administration is a critical aspect of medication management, ensuring that patients receive the appropriate amount of medication for their condition while minimizing the risk of adverse effects. Proper dosage administration involves accurate measurement, appropriate timing, and adherence to the prescribed regimen. Here is an overview of dosage administration:

3.2.1 Key Principles of Dosage Administration

- Carefully review the prescription instructions provided by your healthcare provider. Understand the medication name, dosage, frequency, and any specific administration instructions.
- Use proper measuring tools, such as syringes, droppers, or measuring cups, to ensure precise dosage. Avoid using household spoons, which may not provide accurate measurements.
- Some medications are weight-based or require specific calculations. Always consult your healthcare provider or pharmacist for clarification on the correct dosage.
- Take medications at the specified times to maintain consistent blood levels and achieve the desired therapeutic effect. Use reminders if needed.
- Some medications need to be taken with food or on an empty stomach. Follow the instructions provided to optimize absorption and minimize potential interactions.
- Certain medications may have special administration instructions, such as crushing or splitting tablets, shaking suspensions, or applying topical treatments correctly.
- Some medications require a gradual increase in dosage over time. Follow the titration schedule provided by your healthcare provider.

3.2.2 Dosage Forms

Tablets and Capsules: Swallow tablets and capsules whole with water unless otherwise instructed. Some can be divided or crushed, but consult your healthcare provider or pharmacist first.

Liquid Medications: Use a calibrated measuring device to measure liquid medications accurately. Shake the bottle before use if indicated.

Topical Medications: Apply creams, ointments, or patches to clean and dry skin as directed. Wash your hands before and after application.

Injections: If self-administering injections, follow proper techniques and rotate injection sites. Dispose of needles and syringes safely.

Inhalers: Inhale the medication profoundly and hold your breath for the specified duration. Rinse your mouth if indicated to prevent side effects.

3.2.3 Dosage Adjustments and Safety

- Consult your healthcare provider before making any changes to your dosage, even if you believe an adjustment is necessary.
- Some medications require regular monitoring of blood levels or other parameters. Attend follow-up appointments as recommended.
- Inform your healthcare provider of any changes in your health, such as new symptoms, side effects, or weight changes.
- Medication Interactions: Be cautious about potential interactions between different medications. Inform your healthcare provider about all medicines you are taking.
- Strictly adhere to the prescribed dosage and schedule. If you miss a dose, follow the instructions provided by your healthcare provider or pharmacist.
- Accurate dosage administration is essential for achieving optimal treatment outcomes while minimizing the risk of adverse effects. Always follow your healthcare provider's instructions and communicate openly about any concerns or questions regarding medication dosage and administration.

3.3 Potential Side Effects and Interactions

Understanding potential side effects and interactions of medications is crucial for safe and effective healthcare management. Medications can have beneficial and unintended consequences, including side effects and interactions with other medications, foods, or substances. Here is an overview of potential side effects and interactions:

3.3.1 Potential Side Effects

Common Side Effects: Many medications have common side effects that are often mild and temporary, such as nausea, dizziness, headache, and fatigue.

Serious Side Effects: Some medications can cause more severe side effects, including allergic reactions, organ damage, or changes in blood pressure.

Unintended Effects: Some medications may lead to unintended effects, such as weight gain, mood changes, or blood sugar levels.

Drug Dependence: Certain medications, especially those with the potential for abuse (e.g., opioids), can lead to physical or psychological dependence.

Long-Term Effects: Long-term use of some medications may increase the risk of certain conditions, such as osteoporosis or gastrointestinal bleeding.

Adverse Reactions: Report any unexpected or severe side effects to your healthcare provider immediately.

3.3.2 Medication Interactions

Drug-Drug Interactions: Some medications can interact with each other, potentially enhancing or reducing their effects. Inform your healthcare provider about all medicines you are taking, including over-the-counter drugs, supplements, and herbal products.

Food Interactions: Some medications may interact with certain foods or beverages, affecting their absorption or effectiveness. Follow specific instructions provided by your healthcare provider or pharmacist.

Alcohol and Drug Interactions: Alcohol and recreational drugs can interact with medications, potentially leading to harmful effects or reducing their efficacy.

Drug-Food Interactions: Certain foods can affect how medications are absorbed or metabolized. For example, grapefruit juice can interact with certain medications.

Monitoring and Adjustments: Your healthcare provider will consider potential interactions when prescribing medications and may adjust dosages or choose alternative treatments to minimize risks.

Pharmacokinetic Interactions: Some medications affect how the body processes other drugs, potentially leading to changes in blood levels.

3.3.3 Reducing Risks and Addressing Concerns

Before starting a new medication, inform your healthcare provider about any existing health conditions, allergies, or sensitivities.

Consult a pharmacist to understand potential drug interactions and side effects when filling prescriptions.

Maintain an up-to-date list of all medications you take and share it with healthcare providers.

Follow prescribed dosages and attend regular check-ups to monitor your medication response.

Report any unusual symptoms or changes in your health to your healthcare provider promptly.

Understanding potential side effects and interactions empowers you to make informed decisions about your healthcare. Open communication with your healthcare provider and pharmacist and careful medication management help ensure safe and effective treatment.

3.4 Non-Pharmacological Treatments

Non-pharmacological treatments, also known as non-drug or non-medical treatments, encompass a variety of interventions that can be used to manage health conditions without relying solely on medications. These approaches often focus on lifestyle modifications, therapies, and alternative treatments to promote overall well-being and address specific health concerns. Here is an overview of non-pharmacological treatments:

3.4.1 Lifestyle Modifications

Diet and Nutrition: Adopting a balanced and nutritious diet can play a significant role in managing various health conditions, such as heart disease, diabetes, and obesity. Specific diets, such as the Mediterranean or DASH diet, may be recommended for specific conditions.

Exercise and Physical Activity: Regular physical activity can help improve cardiovascular health, manage weight, enhance muscle strength, and promote mental well-being.

Smoking Cessation: Quitting smoking is crucial for reducing the risk of lung diseases, cardiovascular diseases, and various cancers.

Weight Management: Maintaining a healthy weight is essential for overall health and can contribute to managing conditions such as diabetes and joint problems.

Stress Management: Stress reduction techniques such as meditation, yoga, deep breathing, and mindfulness can help manage stress-related health issues.

Sleep Hygiene: Healthy sleep habits can improve sleep quality and address conditions like insomnia.

3.4.2 Therapies and Interventions

Physical Therapy: Physical therapists provide exercises and techniques to improve mobility, strength, and function in individuals with musculoskeletal or neurological conditions.

Occupational Therapy: Occupational therapists help individuals regain or develop skills needed for daily activities after injury or illness.

Speech Therapy: Speech therapists assist individuals with communication and swallowing difficulties caused by conditions like stroke or neurological disorders.

Cognitive-Behavioral Therapy (CBT): CBT is a psychotherapy approach to address mental health issues such as depression, anxiety, and insomnia.

Physical Modalities: Therapies like heat therapy, cold therapy, ultrasound, and electrical stimulation can relieve pain and promote healing.

Acupuncture: Acupuncture involves inserting thin needles into specific points on the body to promote pain relief and improve overall well-being.

3.4.3 Complementary and Alternative Medicine (CAM)

Herbal Supplements: Certain herbs and botanicals are used for various health purposes, but their safety and efficacy should be discussed with healthcare providers.

Mind-Body Practices: Meditation, yoga, tai chi, and qigong focus on connecting the mind and body to promote relaxation and wellness.

Massage Therapy: Massage can help relieve muscle tension, improve circulation, and reduce stress.

Chiropractic Care: Chiropractors use spinal manipulation and adjustments to address musculoskeletal issues.

Homeopathy: A system of alternative medicine based on the principle of "like cures like," using highly diluted substances to stimulate the body's self-healing abilities.

3.4.4 Patient Education and Self-Management

Patient Counseling: Education and counseling sessions with healthcare professionals can help patients better understand their conditions and make informed decisions about their care.

Self-Monitoring: Regular monitoring of health parameters, such as blood sugar levels or blood pressure, empowers individuals to manage their conditions more effectively.

Self-Care Practices: Learning techniques for wound care, managing chronic conditions, and recognizing symptoms can improve individuals' ability to care for themselves.

Non-pharmacological treatments are often used alone or in combination with medications to provide holistic care and address health's physical, psychological, and emotional aspects. It is essential to consult with healthcare professionals before making significant changes to your treatment plan and to ensure that non-pharmacological treatments are safe and appropriate for your specific condition.

3.5 Surgical Procedures and Aftercare

Surgical procedures are medical interventions that involve the use of instruments and techniques to treat various health conditions by altering or removing tissue, organs, or structures within the body. After undergoing surgery, proper post-operative care and follow-up are essential for a successful recovery. Here is an overview of surgical procedures and aftercare:

3.5.1 Surgical Procedures

Preoperative Assessment: Before surgery, healthcare providers conduct a thorough evaluation to assess the patient's overall health, medical history, and any potential risks associated with the procedure.

Anesthesia: Anesthesia is administered to ensure the patient is comfortable and pain-free during the surgery. Types of anesthesia include general anesthesia (the patient is unconscious), local anesthesia (the specific area is numb), and regional anesthesia (the larger area is numb).

Surgical Techniques: Surgical procedures can be minimally invasive (small incisions using specialized instruments) or open (larger incisions). Surgical techniques vary depending on the specific condition being treated.

Inpatient vs. Outpatient: Some surgeries require hospitalization, while others can be performed on an outpatient basis, allowing the patient to return home the same day.

Recovery Room: After surgery, patients are monitored in a recovery room until they wake up from anesthesia and their vital signs stabilize.

3.5.2 Post-Operative Care and Aftercare

Pain Management: Adequate pain control is essential for patient comfort and recovery. Medications or other pain relief methods are administered as needed.

Wound Care: Proper care of surgical incisions or wounds helps prevent infection and promote healing. Follow healthcare provider instructions for cleaning, dressing changes, and keeping the area dry.

Activity and Mobility: Gradually resume activity and movement as healthcare providers advise. Follow guidelines to prevent straining the surgical site.

Diet and Hydration: Follow dietary instructions, especially if specific restrictions are recommended after surgery. Staying hydrated is essential for recovery.

Medications: Take prescribed medications as directed, including pain relievers, antibiotics, and other medications needed for recovery.

Follow-Up Appointments: Attend follow-up appointments as scheduled to monitor healing progress and address any concerns.

Physical Therapy: Depending on the surgery, physical therapy may be recommended to aid recovery and restore mobility.

Complication Awareness: Be aware of signs of complications such as infection, bleeding, fever, or worsening pain. Promptly report any concerns to healthcare providers.

Emotional Support: Surgery can be physically and emotionally challenging. Seek emotional support from loved ones or consider counseling if needed.

Smoking and Alcohol: Avoid smoking and alcohol during recovery, as they can interfere with healing and increase the risk of complications.

Returning to Normal Activities: Follow healthcare provider instructions on when it is safe to resume normal activities, including work, exercise, and driving.

Each surgical procedure and patient's recovery experience is unique. Adhering to post-operative care instructions and following healthcare provider guidance is essential for a successful and smooth recovery. Proper aftercare helps minimize complications and ensures the best possible outcome from the surgical intervention.

4. Lifestyle and Wellness

4.1 Nutrition and Diet Management

Nutrition and diet management are crucial in promoting overall health and wellness. A balanced and healthy diet provides the necessary nutrients for the body to function optimally and helps prevent or manage various health conditions. Here is an overview of nutrition and diet management:

4.1.1 Key Principles of Nutrition

- Aim to consume various foods from all food groups, including fruits, vegetables, whole grains, lean proteins, and healthy fats.
- Be mindful of portion sizes to avoid overeating. Use tools like measuring cups or visual cues to estimate portion sizes.
- Drink an adequate amount of water throughout the day to stay hydrated. Water is essential for digestion, metabolism, and overall bodily functions.
- Choose nutrient-dense foods that are rich in vitamins, minerals, and antioxidants. These include colorful fruits, vegetables, whole grains, nuts, and lean proteins.
- Reduce consumption of highly processed foods with added sugars, salt, and unhealthy fats.
- Include high-fiber foods such as whole grains, legumes, fruits, and vegetables to support digestion and promote satiety.
- Incorporate sources of healthy fats, such as avocados, nuts, seeds, and fatty fish, which benefit heart health and brain function.

4.1.2 Dietary Considerations for Specific Conditions

- Consume a diet low in saturated and trans fats, sodium, and added sugars. Focus on foods rich in fiber, omega-3 fatty acids, and antioxidants.

- Monitor carbohydrate intake, choose complex carbohydrates, and prioritize foods with a low glycemic index. Balance meals with lean proteins and healthy fats.
- Create a calorie balance by consuming the appropriate calories for your goals. Focus on portion control and a well-balanced diet.
- Ensure sufficient calcium and vitamin D intake through dairy products, leafy greens, and fortified foods.
- Include high-fiber foods and stay hydrated to support regular bowel movements and a healthy gut.

4.1.3 Tips for Healthy Eating

- Plan meals and snacks ahead of time to make nutritious choices and avoid impulsive eating.
- Pay attention to hunger and fullness cues, and eat slowly to savor the flavors and enjoy your meals.
- Consider options like intermittent fasting, mindful eating, or eating smaller, more frequent meals, depending on your preferences and health goals.
- Preparing meals at home allows you to control ingredients and portion sizes.
- Learn to read nutrition labels to make informed choices about packaged foods.
- Choose water, herbal teas, or unsweetened beverages over sugary drinks.
- Enjoy treats and less nutritious foods in moderation rather than as a regular diet.
- Consult a registered dietitian or nutritionist for personalized dietary recommendations tailored to your health needs and goals.

Nutrition and diet management are essential components of a healthy lifestyle. Making informed food choices and adopting a balanced diet can positively impact your well-being, energy levels, and overall health. Remember that individual dietary needs may vary, so working with healthcare professionals to create a nutrition plan that suits your needs and goals is essential.

4.2 Physical Activity and Exercise Guidelines

Physical activity and exercise are integral to maintaining good health, improving fitness, and preventing various health conditions. Regular physical activity offers numerous benefits for both the body and mind. Here is an overview of physical activity and exercise guidelines:

4.2.1 Importance of Physical Activity

Cardiovascular Health: Regular exercise helps improve heart health by increasing cardiovascular fitness, reducing the risk of heart disease, and lowering blood pressure.

Weight Management: Physical activity contributes to weight loss and maintenance by burning calories and increasing metabolism.

Muscle Strength and Endurance: Exercise promotes muscle development, strength, and endurance, enhancing overall physical performance.

Bone Health: Weight-bearing activities like walking, running, and resistance training help maintain bone density and reduce the risk of osteoporosis.

Mental Well-Being: Physical activity reduces stress, anxiety, and depression, promoting overall well-being.

Blood Sugar Control: Regular exercise can help manage blood sugar levels and reduce the risk of type 2 diabetes.

Improved Sleep: Physical activity can improve sleep quality and duration, leading to better rest and recovery.

4.2.2 Physical Activity Guidelines

Aerobic Activity: Aim for at least 150 minutes of moderate-intensity aerobic activity (e.g., brisk walking, cycling) per week or 75 minutes of vigorous-intensity aerobic activity (e.g., running, swimming).

Muscle-Strengthening: Include muscle-strengthening activities targeting major muscle groups two or more days per week. This can involve weight lifting, bodyweight exercises, or resistance bands.

Flexibility and Balance: Incorporate activities that improve flexibility, such as stretching, and exercises that enhance balance, especially for older adults.

4.2.3 Exercise Considerations

- If you are new to exercise, start with low-intensity activities and gradually increase the duration and intensity.
- Always begin with a warm-up to prepare your body for exercise and end with a cool-down to gradually decrease your heart rate.
- Include a mix of aerobic, strength, and flexibility exercises to target different aspects of fitness.
- Pay attention to how your body responds to exercise. Rest and recover when needed, and consult a healthcare provider if you experience pain or discomfort.
- Drink water before, during, and after exercise to stay hydrated, especially in hot or humid conditions.
- Wear comfortable and appropriate clothing and footwear for your chosen activity.
- Consult a healthcare provider before starting a new exercise program if you have existing health conditions or concerns.

4.2.4 Staying Motivated

- Establish clear, achievable fitness goals to stay motivated and track progress.

- ❖ Try different types of exercise to prevent boredom and keep things interesting.
- ❖ Choose activities you like to increase the likelihood of sticking with them long-term.
- ❖ Exercise with friends, join group classes or participate in sports to make physical activity more enjoyable.
- ❖ Keep a workout journal or use fitness apps to monitor your progress and celebrate achievements.

Physical activity is a powerful tool for maintaining health and wellness. By incorporating regular exercise into your routine, you can enjoy a healthier lifestyle, improved fitness, and a better quality of life. Always consult a healthcare provider before beginning a new exercise program, especially if you have any pre-existing health conditions or concerns.

4.3 Stress Management and Mental Health

Stress management and mental health are vital components of overall well-being. The demands of modern life can contribute to stress, anxiety, and other mental health challenges. Adopting effective strategies for managing stress and promoting mental wellness is essential for maintaining a balanced and healthy lifestyle. Here is an overview of stress management and mental health:

4.3.1 Understanding Stress

Types of Stress: Stress can be acute (short-term) or chronic (long-term). Acute stress is a normal response to challenging situations, while chronic stress can negatively affect physical and mental health.

Impact of Stress: Prolonged stress can lead to various health issues, including cardiovascular problems, weakened immune systems, sleep disturbances, and mood disorders.

4.3.2 Stress Management Strategies

Mindfulness and Meditation: Mindfulness and meditation techniques can help you stay present, reduce anxiety, and manage stress.

Deep Breathing: Deep breathing exercises can help calm the nervous system and reduce stress responses.

Physical Activity: Regular exercise is a powerful stress reliever, promoting the release of endorphins and improving mood.

Healthy Lifestyle: Prioritize balanced nutrition, adequate sleep, and regular physical activity to support overall well-being.

Time Management: Organize your tasks, set priorities, and create a schedule to manage daily responsibilities effectively.

Social Support: Spend time with supportive friends and family members who can provide encouragement and understanding.

Hobbies and Activities: Engage in hobbies and activities you enjoy to take a break from stressors and promote relaxation.

4.3.3 Mental Health and Well-Being

- ❖ Prioritize self-care activities that bring you joy and relaxation, such as reading, walking, or practicing hobbies.
- ❖ Cultivate positive relationships and open communication with loved ones.
- ❖ If you are experiencing persistent stress, anxiety, or other mental health concerns, consider seeking support from a mental health professional, such as a counselor or therapist.
- ❖ Reduce exposure to negative news, social media, and other stress-inducing sources.
- ❖ Develop a growth mindset by focusing on solutions and viewing challenges as opportunities for personal growth.

- Regularly expressing gratitude for positive aspects of your life can improve your overall well-being.

4.3.4 Seeking Help

- Be aware of signs of stress or mental health challenges, such as changes in sleep patterns, mood swings, persistent worry, or social withdrawal.
- Reach out to a trusted friend, family member, or professional if you need to discuss your feelings or concerns.
- If stress or mental health symptoms become overwhelming, consider seeking guidance from a mental health professional. Therapists, counselors, and psychiatrists can provide personalized strategies and support.

Prioritizing stress management and mental health practices can significantly improve your quality of life, enhance resilience, and contribute to a more balanced and upbeat lifestyle. Remember that seeking Help is a sign of strength, and taking steps to care for your mental well-being is a valuable investment in your overall health.

4.4 Sleep Hygiene and Restful Practices

Sleep hygiene and restful practices are essential for maintaining optimal health and well-being. Quality sleep is crucial for physical, mental, and emotional health. Adopting healthy sleep habits and creating a relaxing sleep environment can improve sleep quality and overall wellness. Here is an overview of sleep hygiene and restful practices:

4.4.1 Importance of Sleep

- Sleep allows the body to repair and regenerate tissues, promote muscle growth, and support immune function.
- Quality sleep is essential for cognitive function, memory consolidation, and emotional well-being.

- ❖ Adequate sleep helps boost energy levels, concentration, and productivity during waking hours.
- ❖ Sleep plays a role in regulating hormones that control appetite, stress, and growth.

4.4.2 Sleep Hygiene Practices

Consistent Schedule: Go to bed and wake up simultaneously every day, even on weekends, to regulate your body's internal clock.

Create a Sleep-Friendly Environment:

- ➢ Keep your bedroom dark, quiet, and at a comfortable temperature.
- ➢ Use a comfortable mattress and pillows that provide adequate support.
- ➢ Minimize noise and distractions that could disrupt sleep.

Limit Screen Time: Avoid electronic devices (phones, tablets, computers) before bedtime, as the blue light emitted can interfere with melatonin production and disrupt sleep.

Relaxation Routine: Engage in calming activities before bed, such as reading, practicing gentle yoga, or taking a warm bath.

Limit Stimulants: Avoid caffeine and nicotine close to bedtime, as they can interfere with falling asleep.

Regular Physical Activity: Engage in regular exercise, but avoid vigorous activity close to bedtime.

Mindful Eating: Avoid heavy, spicy, or large meals before bedtime. A light snack may be preferable if you are hungry.

Alcohol and Sleep: Limit alcohol consumption, as it can disrupt sleep patterns and lead to fragmented sleep.

4.4.3 Restful Practices

Mindfulness Meditation: Engage in mindfulness meditation or deep breathing exercises to promote relaxation and reduce stress before bed.

Progressive Muscle Relaxation: Tense each muscle group to induce relaxation.

Aromatherapy: Use calming scents like lavender through essential oils, diffusers, or sprays.

White Noise or Relaxing Sounds: Play calming sounds like nature sounds, white noise, or soothing music to create a peaceful sleep environment.

Journaling: Write down your thoughts, worries, or gratitudes before bed to clear your mind and promote a sense of closure.

Visualization: Imagine yourself in a peaceful and relaxing setting to encourage relaxation.

Limit Napping: If you nap during the day, keep it short (20-30 minutes) and avoid napping too close to bedtime.

4.4.4 Seeking Help for Sleep Issues

If you experience persistent sleep difficulties, such as insomnia, consider seeking guidance from a healthcare provider or sleep specialist.

If you suspect a sleep disorder (e.g., sleep apnea, restless legs syndrome), consult a healthcare professional for evaluation and management.

Prioritizing sleep hygiene and adopting restful practices can profoundly impact your overall well-being. By creating a sleep-friendly environment and incorporating relaxation techniques into your routine, you can enhance your sleep quality and enjoy the numerous benefits of restorative rest.

4.5 Substance Abuse Prevention and Cessation

Substance abuse prevention and cessation are crucial to a healthy lifestyle and overall wellness. Substance abuse, including the misuse of alcohol, tobacco, prescription medications, and illicit drugs, can seriously negatively affect physical and mental health. Adopting strategies to prevent substance abuse and seeking cessation help can improve well-being and quality of life. Here is an overview of substance abuse prevention and cessation:

4.5.1 Substance Abuse Prevention

- ❖ Stay informed about the risks and consequences of substance abuse through reliable sources of information.
- ❖ Identify and address risk factors or signs of substance abuse in yourself or others, and seek help early.
- ❖ Develop healthy ways to cope with stress, anxiety, and other emotions, such as exercise, mindfulness, and social support.
- ❖ Practice assertiveness skills to resist peer pressure and make confident decisions that align with your values.
- ❖ Surround yourself with supportive friends and engage in social activities that do not involve substance use.
- ❖ Parents and caregivers can significantly prevent substance abuse by communicating openly with their children and setting clear expectations.

4.5.2 Substance Cessation

- ❖ If you are struggling with substance abuse, contact a healthcare provider, counselor, or addiction specialist for guidance and support.

- ❖ Certain medications, counseling, and behavioral therapies can aid in substance use disorder treatment.
- ❖ Participate in counseling and behavioral therapies tailored to address the underlying causes of substance abuse and develop coping skills.
- ❖ Join support groups or 12-step programs that provide a sense of community and understanding from others who have experienced similar challenges.
- ❖ Surround yourself with people who encourage your recovery and distance yourself from those who may enable substance use.
- ❖ Learn mindfulness techniques and stress reduction strategies to manage triggers and cravings.

4.5.3 Alcohol and Tobacco Cessation

Alcohol Moderation or Abstinence: If you choose to drink alcohol, do so in moderation. For those struggling with alcohol dependence, complete abstinence may be necessary.

Tobacco Cessation: Quitting smoking or using tobacco products significantly improves health. Explore nicotine replacement therapies, medications, and counseling to support cessation.

4.5.4 Prescription Medication Safety

- ➢ Take prescription medications as prescribed and discuss any concerns or side effects with your healthcare provider.
- ➢ Do not share prescription medications with others, and avoid taking medications not prescribed to you.

4.5.5 Illicit Drugs

Do not use illicit drugs, which can have serious health risks and legal consequences.

If you are using illicit drugs, seek Help from a healthcare professional or addiction specialist to explore treatment options.

Prioritizing substance abuse prevention and cessation is essential to improving your overall health and well-being. If you or someone you know is struggling with substance abuse, remember that seeking Help and support is a sign of strength, and resources are available to guide you on the path to recovery.

5. Special Patient Groups

5.1 Pediatrics and Childcare

Pediatrics and childcare involve specialized care for infants, children, and adolescents to ensure their growth, development, and well-being. Proper pediatric care encompasses a range of medical, developmental, and emotional considerations. Here is an overview of pediatrics and childcare:

5.1.1 Well-Baby and Well-Child Visits

Regular Check-ups: Pediatricians monitor a child's growth, development, and overall health through regular well-baby and well-child visits.

Vaccinations: Vaccinations are essential to pediatric care to protect children from preventable diseases.

Developmental Milestones: Pediatricians assess a child's milestones, such as motor skills, speech, and social development, to ensure they progress appropriately.

Nutrition: Pediatricians guide infant feeding, introducing solid foods and maintaining a balanced diet as children grow.

5.1.2 Common Pediatric Health Concerns

Infections: Children are prone to common infections such as colds, ear infections, and respiratory infections.

Allergies: Pediatricians diagnose and manage allergies, including food and allergic reactions.

Asthma: Asthma management involves monitoring symptoms, using inhalers, and creating an asthma action plan.

Skin Conditions: Pediatricians address skin issues like eczema, rashes, and acne in children.

Behavioral and Developmental Issues: Pediatricians assess and provide interventions for behavioral concerns, attention disorders, and developmental delays.

5.1.3 Parenting and Childcare

- ❖ A robust parent-child bond is essential for a child's emotional development and well-being.
- ❖ Educate parents on safe sleep practices to reduce the risk of Sudden Infant Death Syndrome (SIDS).
- ❖ Teach parents about childproofing their home, using car seats, and preventing accidents.
- ❖ Provide strategies for positive discipline and managing challenging behaviors.
- ❖ Offer guidance for supporting children's emotional needs and addressing anxiety or stress.

5.1.4 Adolescents and Teenagers

- ❖ Provide accurate information about puberty, sexual health, and safe practices.
- ❖ Address mental health concerns such as depression, anxiety, and stress that often arise during adolescence.
- ❖ Educate teenagers about the risks of substance abuse and provide guidance on making healthy choices.
- ❖ Discuss healthy relationship dynamics, communication, and consent.
- ❖ Address body image concerns and promote self-confidence and positive self-esteem.

Pediatrics and childcare involve a holistic approach encompassing medical care, developmental monitoring, and parental guidance. Regular well-child visits, open communication with healthcare providers, and a supportive home environment contribute to optimal growth, development, and well-being for children and adolescents.

5.2 Geriatrics and Aging Healthfully

Geriatrics focuses on the medical care and well-being of older adults, commonly called geriatric patients. As people age, their healthcare needs and considerations change, and specialized care is essential to promote healthy aging. Here is an overview of geriatrics and aging healthfully:

5.2.1 Health Considerations in Geriatrics

Chronic Conditions: Geriatric patients often have multiple chronic conditions such as hypertension, diabetes, heart disease, and arthritis. Managing these conditions is a crucial aspect of geriatric care.

Polypharmacy: Older adults may be prescribed multiple medications, increasing the risk of interactions and side effects. Medication management is crucial.

Cognitive Health: Assess and monitor cognitive function, memory, and risk factors for conditions like Alzheimer's disease and other forms of dementia.

Functional Decline: Address physical and functional changes accompanying aging, such as mobility issues, balance problems, and falls.

Nutritional Needs: Address changing nutritional needs and dietary considerations for older adults to maintain optimal health.

5.2.2 Comprehensive Geriatric Assessment

- ❖ A thorough physical assessment helps identify health concerns and develop an individualized care plan.
- ❖ Evaluate memory, cognition, and mental health to detect early signs of cognitive decline.
- ❖ Review and optimize medication regimens to minimize side effects and interactions.
- ❖ Assess daily living activities, mobility, and physical function to determine independence and support needs.
- ❖ Address psychological well-being, depression, loneliness, and social support to improve the overall quality of life.

5.2.3 Age-Related Health Promotion

- ❖ Encourage regular exercise to maintain muscle strength, bone density, and cardiovascular health.
- ❖ Emphasize a balanced diet of nutrients to support energy levels and prevent malnutrition.
- ❖ Address osteoporosis prevention and management through calcium and vitamin D intake, weight-bearing exercise, and medication if needed.
- ❖ Implement strategies to prevent falls, such as home modifications, balance exercises, and regular vision checks.
- ❖ Engage in cognitive activities, puzzles, and social interactions to promote brain health.

5.2.4 Palliative and Hospice Care

Palliative Care: Focus on relieving symptoms and improving the quality of life for individuals with serious illnesses.

Hospice Care: Offer compassionate end-of-life care and support for terminally ill individuals and their families.

5.2.5 Mental and Emotional Health

- ❖ Address mental health concerns and provide appropriate interventions, including therapy or medication.
- ❖ Encourage social activities, clubs, and support groups to combat feelings of isolation and loneliness.
- ❖ Discuss and document medical treatment and end-of-life care preferences.

Geriatrics emphasizes personalized care that promotes healthy aging, maintains independence, and enhances the quality of life for older adults. Regular healthcare check-ups, open communication with healthcare providers, and focusing on physical, emotional, and cognitive well-being contribute to successful aging.

5.3 Pregnancy, Prenatal Care, and Postpartum Support

Pregnancy, prenatal care, and postpartum support are critical stages in a woman's life that require specialized care to ensure the health and well-being of both the mother and the baby. Proper care and support during these stages contribute to a healthy pregnancy, safe childbirth, and a smooth transition to motherhood. Here is an overview of pregnancy, prenatal care, and postpartum support:

5.3.1 Pregnancy and Prenatal Care

- ❖ Regular prenatal check-ups with a healthcare provider are essential to monitor the health of both the mother and the developing fetus.
- ❖ Educate pregnant women about proper nutrition, balanced diets, and prenatal vitamins to support the baby's growth and development.
- ❖ Encourage safe and appropriate exercise during pregnancy to maintain physical fitness and reduce discomfort.

- ❖ Utilize ultrasounds and other tests to monitor the baby's growth, development, and overall health.
- ❖ Address common pregnancy discomforts such as nausea, back pain, and fatigue through lifestyle adjustments and interventions.

5.3.2 Labor and Childbirth

Labor Education: Provide childbirth education classes to prepare expectant parents for labor, delivery, and postpartum care.

Labor Support: Offer options for pain relief and comfort measures during labor, including epidurals, breathing techniques, and movement.

Delivery Options: Discuss various delivery options, including vaginal birth, cesarean section, and assisted delivery.

5.3.3 Postpartum Support

Physical Recovery: Support postpartum healing and recovery, including managing postpartum pain and addressing physical changes.

Breastfeeding Support: Offer guidance on breastfeeding techniques, positioning, and addressing common breastfeeding challenges.

Mental Health: Monitor and support postpartum mood disorders such as postpartum depression and anxiety.

Newborn Care: Educate parents about newborn care, including feeding, diapering, and safe sleep practices.

Family Support: Engage partners and family members in postpartum care and encourage open communication.

5.3.4 Family Planning and Contraception

Birth Control Options: Discuss contraception methods and family planning to help individuals make informed decisions about their reproductive health.

Postpartum Contraception: Address options for birth control after childbirth, considering breastfeeding and individual health factors.

5.3.5 Preparing for Another Pregnancy

Discuss optimal timing for subsequent pregnancies, address health concerns, and optimize maternal and fetal well-being.

5.3.6 Genetic Counseling

Provide genetic counseling and testing for couples with a history of genetic disorders or family concerns.

Proper prenatal care and postpartum support are essential for the mother's and newborn's health and well-being. Tailored guidance, education, and monitoring throughout pregnancy and postpartum contribute to a positive pregnancy experience and a healthy start for the new family.

5.4 Chronic Disease Management

Chronic disease management involves specialized care for individuals with long-term medical conditions. These conditions often require ongoing monitoring, treatment, and lifestyle adjustments to effectively manage symptoms, prevent complications, and maintain quality of life. Here is an overview of chronic disease management:

5.4.1 Understanding Chronic Diseases

Common Chronic Diseases: Chronic diseases include conditions such as diabetes, hypertension (high blood pressure), heart disease, chronic obstructive pulmonary disease (COPD), arthritis, and more.

Long-Term Nature: Chronic diseases are typically ongoing and may require lifelong management to control symptoms and reduce the risk of complications.

Multidisciplinary Approach: Effective chronic disease management often involves a team of healthcare professionals, including doctors, nurses, specialists, dietitians, and mental health professionals.

5.4.2 Chronic Disease Management Strategies

Medication Management: Consistently take prescribed medications as directed and communicate any concerns or side effects to your healthcare provider.

Lifestyle Modifications: Adopt healthy lifestyle habits such as a balanced diet, regular physical activity, smoking cessation, and stress reduction.

Regular Monitoring: Attend scheduled medical appointments to monitor your condition and adjust treatment plans as needed.

Self-Care and Education: Educate yourself about your condition, its management, and potential complications. Engage in self-care practices to manage symptoms.

Goal Setting: Collaborate with your healthcare team to set achievable goals for managing your condition and improving your overall well-being.

Emotional Support: Address the emotional impact of living with a chronic disease through counseling, support groups, and stress management techniques.

5.4.3 Diabetes Management

- Regularly monitor blood glucose levels and adjust insulin or medication doses as needed.
- Follow a balanced diet that manages carbohydrate intake and promotes stable blood sugar levels.
- Regularly exercise to improve insulin sensitivity and support overall health.
- Pay attention to foot health and practice proper foot care to prevent complications.

5.4.4 Cardiovascular Disease Management

- Monitor and manage blood pressure through lifestyle changes and medication.
- Follow guidelines for maintaining healthy cholesterol levels through Diet, exercise, and medication if necessary.
- Adopt a diet low in saturated and trans fats, sodium, and added sugars to support heart health.

5.4.5 COPD Management

- Quit smoking to slow the progression of COPD and improve lung function.
- Learn breathing exercises and techniques to manage breathlessness.
- Take prescribed medications, including bronchodilators and anti-inflammatory drugs, as directed.

Chronic disease management requires a proactive and collaborative approach between patients and healthcare providers. Open communication, adherence to treatment plans, and a focus on healthy lifestyle choices are essential to effectively managing chronic conditions and maintaining a good quality of life. Regular medical check-ups, education, and support systems are crucial in helping individuals successfully manage their chronic diseases.

6. Preventive Care and Screenings

6.1 Immunizations and Vaccination Schedules

Immunizations and vaccinations are essential components of preventive care that protect individuals from various infectious diseases. Vaccinations work by stimulating the immune system to produce antibodies against specific pathogens, helping to prevent illness and the spread of contagious diseases. Here is an overview of immunizations and vaccination schedules:

6.1.1 Importance of Immunizations

Immunizations are a highly effective way to prevent the spread of infectious diseases and reduce the incidence of serious illnesses.

Vaccinations contribute to "herd immunity," which helps protect individuals who cannot be vaccinated, such as those with weakened immune systems or certain medical conditions.

Widespread vaccination reduces the burden on healthcare systems by preventing hospitalizations and medical expenses associated with preventable diseases.

6.1.2 Vaccination Schedules

Childhood Immunizations: Follow the recommended childhood vaccination schedule provided by healthcare providers. This schedule typically includes vaccines for measles, mumps, rubella, polio, diphtheria, tetanus, pertussis, and more.

Adolescent Vaccinations: Certain vaccinations, such as the HPV and meningococcal vaccines, are recommended during adolescence to protect against specific diseases.

Adult Vaccinations: Adults should receive booster doses of certain vaccines and may also require vaccines based on their health status and risk factors. Vaccinations for influenza, pneumococcal disease, and shingles are commonly recommended for older adults.

Travel Vaccines: Individuals traveling to specific regions may need additional vaccinations to protect against diseases that are prevalent in those areas.

6.1.3 Vaccine Safety

Research and Development: Vaccines undergo rigorous safety and effectiveness testing before being approved.

Monitoring: Ongoing monitoring ensures that vaccines remain safe and effective after they are introduced to the population.

Side Effects: Most vaccine side effects, such as soreness at the injection site or a low-grade fever, are mild and temporary. Serious side effects are rare.

Vaccine Myths: Address vaccine misinformation and myths by providing accurate information based on scientific evidence.

6.1.4 Special Considerations

Vaccination During Pregnancy: Some vaccines are recommended for pregnant individuals to protect the mother and the developing baby. These include the flu and Tdap vaccines (tetanus, diphtheria, and pertussis).

Vaccination for Immunocompromised Individuals: Certain individuals with weakened immune systems may need particular vaccination recommendations. Consult with a healthcare provider for guidance.

Catch-Up Vaccination: If a person misses a vaccine dose, catch-up vaccination schedules are available to ensure they receive the necessary protection.

Vaccinations are a cornerstone of preventive medicine, safeguarding individuals and communities from serious and potentially life-threatening diseases. Staying up-to-date with recommended immunizations is vital to maintaining optimal health and preventing the spread of contagious illnesses. It is essential to consult with healthcare providers to determine the appropriate vaccination schedule for you and your family based on age, health status, and individual risk factors.

6.2 Cancer Screenings and Early Detection

Cancer screenings and early detection are crucial in identifying cancer at its earliest and most treatable stages. Regular screenings can significantly improve the chances of successful treatment and positive outcomes. Here is a comprehensive overview of cancer screenings and early detection:

6.2.1 Importance of Cancer Screenings

Cancer screenings aim to catch cancers in their initial stages when treatment is more effective, and outcomes are better.

Regular screenings can lower mortality rates by detecting cancers before they become advanced and harder to treat.

Healthcare providers assess individual risk factors to determine personalized screening recommendations based on age, gender, family history, and lifestyle.

6.2.2 Common Cancer Screenings

Breast Cancer: Mammograms are recommended for women starting around age 40 or earlier with a family history of breast cancer. Clinical breast exams and self-exams also play a role.

Cervical Cancer: Pap smears are used to screen for cervical cancer in women, typically starting at age 21. HPV testing may also be recommended.

Colorectal Cancer: Screening methods include colonoscopy, sigmoidoscopy, and stool tests. Regular screenings usually begin around age 50.

Prostate Cancer: PSA blood tests and digital rectal exams (DRE) are used to screen for prostate cancer in men, usually around age 50.

Lung Cancer: Low-dose computed tomography (LDCT) scans are recommended for individuals at high risk of lung cancer, such as heavy smokers.

6.2.3 Early Detection and Self-Exams

Skin Cancer: Regularly examine your skin for moles and changes, and consult a healthcare provider if you notice anything suspicious.

Testicular Cancer: Men should perform routine testicular self-exams to detect unusual lumps or changes.

Oral Cancer: Dental check-ups may include oral cancer screenings. Be vigilant about mouth sores, patches, or persistent changes.

6.2.4 Screening Guidelines

Age and Frequency: Follow recommended screening guidelines based on age, gender, and risk factors. Discuss screening schedules with healthcare providers.

Informed Decisions: Engage in shared decision-making with healthcare providers to determine the most suitable approach to cancer screenings based on your health and preferences.

Understanding the Process: Familiarize yourself with the benefits and limitations of screenings, including potential false-positive or false-negative results.

6.2.5 Follow-Up and Treatment

Diagnostic Tests: Additional diagnostic tests like biopsies or imaging may be recommended if a screening test raises concerns.

Timely Intervention: If cancer is detected, prompt treatment can improve outcomes and lead to a cure.

Holistic Support: Access support services, including counseling and support groups, to navigate a cancer diagnosis and treatment's emotional and physical challenges.

Participating in cancer screenings and prioritizing early detection are fundamental steps in maintaining your health. By adhering to recommended screening guidelines and collaborating with healthcare providers, you can take proactive measures to catch cancer in its earliest stages and receive timely and effective interventions.

6.3 Routine Health Check-ups and Monitoring

Routine health check-ups and monitoring are essential components of preventive care that help individuals maintain their overall well-being and identify potential health issues early. Regular visits to healthcare providers allow for the assessment of health status, the management of chronic conditions, and the implementation of preventive measures. Here is an overview of routine health check-ups and monitoring

6.3.1 Importance of Routine Check-ups

- ❖ Regular health check-ups facilitate the early detection of health problems, enabling timely intervention and treatment.
- ❖ Check-ups allow healthcare providers to offer personalized preventive recommendations based on individual health risks and needs.
- ❖ Routine visits promote healthy behaviors, lifestyle modifications, and overall well-being.

6.3.2 Components of Routine Check-ups

Physical Examination: Healthcare providers perform a comprehensive physical assessment to evaluate general health, vital signs, and potential concerns.

Medical History Review: Discuss any changes in health, medications, symptoms, or lifestyle since the last visit.

Screenings and Tests: Depending on age, gender, and risk factors, screenings for conditions such as blood pressure, cholesterol, diabetes, and cancer may be conducted.

Immunizations: Ensure that immunizations are up-to-date based on age and recommended schedules.

Nutritional Counseling: Receive guidance on maintaining a balanced diet and making healthy food choices.

Lifestyle Recommendations: Healthcare providers offer advice on exercise, stress management, sleep, and other lifestyle factors.

Medication Review: Discuss current medications, adherence, and potential interactions.

6.3.3 Monitoring Chronic Conditions

- Regular check-ups are crucial for individuals with chronic conditions to monitor disease progression and optimize management.
- Healthcare providers may adjust medications or treatment plans based on monitoring results.
- Early identification and intervention can prevent complications and improve the quality of life for those with chronic conditions.

6.3.4 Age-Related Considerations

Pediatrics: Children require regular well-child visits to monitor growth, development, and immunizations.

Adolescents: Routine visits for adolescents focus on growth, mental health, preventive measures, and counseling.

Adults: Routine check-ups involve health maintenance, preventive screenings, and age-specific health concerns.

Seniors: Geriatric assessments address age-related health considerations, cognitive function, and chronic disease management.

6.3.5 Follow-Up and Communication

- Healthcare providers create personalized action plans, including lifestyle changes, referrals, or further tests.
- Openly discuss any health concerns or questions with healthcare providers during check-ups.
- Keep track of personal health records, including test results, medications, and treatment plans.

Routine health check-ups and monitoring are essential for maintaining good health, preventing potential issues, and receiving timely medical attention. By actively participating in regular visits to healthcare providers and following their recommendations, individuals can take proactive steps toward preserving their well-being and enjoying a higher quality of life.

7. Health Resources and Support

7.1 Accessing Healthcare Services

Accessing healthcare services is a crucial aspect of maintaining your health and well-being. Access to quality medical care ensures timely prevention, diagnosis, and treatment of health conditions. Here is an overview of how to access healthcare services effectively:

7.1.1 Primary Care Providers

- ❖ Choose a Primary Care Physician (PCP) who will be your main point of contact for general healthcare needs, routine check-ups, and referrals to specialists.
- ❖ Schedule routine appointments with your PCP for preventive care and health maintenance.
- ❖ Establish clear communication with your PCP, share your medical history, and discuss any concerns you may have.

7.1.2 Specialists

If needed, your PCP may refer you to specialists for specific health concerns or conditions.

Consult with specialists for in-depth evaluations, second opinions, and specialized treatments.

7.1.3 Urgent Care and Emergency Services

Visit urgent care centers for non-life-threatening illnesses or injuries requiring prompt attention but not emergencies.

In emergencies, such as severe injuries or life-threatening conditions, seek care at an emergency room or call emergency services.

7.1.4 Telehealth Services

Take advantage of telehealth services for remote consultations with healthcare providers for minor concerns, follow-up appointments, and prescription refills.

7.1.5 Health Insurance

Obtain health insurance coverage to help manage medical care, prescriptions, and preventive services costs.

Familiarize yourself with your health insurance policy, including deductibles, copayments, and covered services.

Choose healthcare providers and facilities within your insurance network to maximize coverage and minimize out-of-pocket costs.

7.1.6 Community Health Centers

Access community health centers that offer affordable healthcare services to individuals and families, including those without insurance.

Community health centers often provide vaccinations, screenings, and wellness programs.

7.1.7 Prescription Medications

If you have prescription coverage, fill your prescriptions at pharmacies within your insurance network to save on costs.

Opt for generic medications, when possible, as they are often more cost-effective.

Take medications as prescribed and discuss any concerns or side effects with your healthcare provider.

7.1.8 Patient Portals and Apps

Utilize patient portals and healthcare apps to schedule appointments, view test results, and communicate with your healthcare team.

7.1.9 Health Education and Support

Seek reliable health information from reputable sources, including government websites, medical organizations, and healthcare providers.

Join support groups for specific health conditions to connect with others facing similar challenges.

Accessing healthcare services involves understanding your options, seeking timely care, and utilizing available resources. By establishing a healthcare relationship, staying informed, and utilizing various avenues of care, you can prioritize your health and well-being effectively.

7.2 Health Insurance and Financial Assistance

Health insurance and financial assistance play crucial roles in ensuring access to quality healthcare services and managing the costs associated with medical care. Understanding health insurance options and available financial support can help individuals and families navigate the healthcare system more effectively. Here is an overview of health insurance and financial assistance:

7.2.1 Health Insurance Options

Many employers offer health insurance plans to their employees and their families health insurance plans of coverage options.

If an employer does not cover you, you can purchase individual health insurance plans through state or federal marketplaces or directly from insurance providers.

Medicaid provides health coverage to eligible low-income individuals and families. Eligibility and benefits vary by state.

Medicare is a federal health insurance program for individuals aged 65 and older and specifically younger individuals with disabilities.

COBRA allows individuals to continue their employer-sponsored health insurance coverage for a limited period after leaving their job.

7.2.2 Understanding Health Insurance

Understand your health insurance plan's coverage and benefits, including deductibles, copayments, coinsurance, and covered services.

Choose healthcare providers and facilities within your insurance network to maximize coverage and minimize out-of-pocket costs.

Many health insurance plans cover preventive services such as vaccinations, screenings, and annual check-ups at no cost to the insured.

7.2.3 Financial Assistance and Support

Depending on your income and family size, you may qualify for subsidies or premium tax credits that reduce the cost of health insurance premiums.

Some states have expanded Medicaid eligibility, providing coverage to more low-income individuals and families.

Health Savings Accounts (HSAs) and Flexible Spending Accounts (FSAs) allow you to set aside pre-tax money to pay for eligible medical expenses.

Many pharmaceutical companies offer patient assistance programs with discounts or free medications to needy individuals.

Charitable and nonprofit organizations offer financial assistance or grants to help cover medical costs for specific conditions.

7.2.4 Applying for Financial Assistance

Enroll in health insurance plans through state or federal marketplaces during open enrollment periods.

Apply for Medicaid or the Children's Health Insurance Program (CHIP) through your state's Medicaid agency.

Enroll in Medicare when you become eligible based on age or disability status.

Research and apply for financial assistance programs that can help cover medical costs.

7.2.5 Managing Costs

Plan for medical expenses by including them in your budget and setting aside funds for deductibles, copayments, and other out-of-pocket costs.

If you receive a medical bill you cannot afford, contact the healthcare provider to discuss payment options or negotiate the bill.

Contact your health insurance provider to understand your coverage and costs before receiving medical services.

Navigating health insurance and seeking financial assistance can be complex, but it is crucial for accessing necessary healthcare services. By exploring available options, understanding your coverage, and taking advantage of financial assistance programs, you can ensure that you and your family receive the care you need without facing overwhelming financial burdens.

7.3 Patient Advocacy and Support Groups

Patient advocacy and support groups are vital in providing emotional, informational, and practical assistance to individuals facing medical challenges. These resources offer community, education, and empowerment for patients and their families. Here is an overview of patient advocacy and support groups.

7.3.1 Patient Advocacy

Definition: Patient advocates are individuals or organizations that work on behalf of patients to ensure they receive the best possible care and support.

Roles of Patient Advocates:

a. Navigating the Healthcare System: Patient advocates help patients understand their diagnoses, treatment options, and medical bills.
b. Communication: Advocates facilitate communication between patients, families, and healthcare providers.
c. Education: Advocates provide information about medical conditions, treatments, and resources.
d. Rights and Privacy: Advocates ensure patient rights and privacy are respected.

Professional Patient Advocates: Some individuals work as professional patient advocates, offering their expertise to guide patients through medical decisions and interactions.

7.3.2 Support Groups

Definition: Support groups bring together individuals with similar health conditions, experiences, or challenges to provide mutual support and information.

Benefits of Support Groups:

a. Emotional Support: Connecting with others who understand your experiences can alleviate feelings of isolation and provide emotional comfort.
b. Information Sharing: Support groups offer a platform to exchange information, resources, and coping strategies.
c. Empowerment: Participating in a support group can empower individuals to take an active role in their healthcare journey.

7.3.3 Types of Support Groups

Condition-Specific Groups: These groups focus on a particular medical condition, such as cancer, diabetes, or autoimmune diseases.

Caregiver Support Groups: Caregiver groups offer assistance and emotional support for those caring for loved ones with medical needs.

Online Support Communities: Virtual platforms allow individuals to connect and share experiences online.

7.3.4 How to Access Patient Advocacy and Support

Ask your healthcare provider or clinic about local patient advocacy resources and support groups.

Explore reputable websites and organizations related to your condition or needs.

Search for online support groups or patient advocacy communities on social media platforms.

Check with local hospitals, community centers, or nonprofit organizations for information on support groups.

7.3.5 Participation and Benefits

Active Participation: Discuss, attend meetings, and share your experiences to contribute to the support group community.

Emotional Well-Being: Connecting with others facing similar challenges can improve your emotional well-being and reduce feelings of loneliness.

Learning and Coping: Support groups provide a platform to learn about your condition, treatments, and effective coping strategies.

Empowerment: Interacting with patient advocates and support group members can empower you to make informed healthcare decisions.

Patient advocacy and support groups create a network of understanding and compassion, fostering community and empowerment among individuals facing medical challenges. By connecting with these resources, you can gain valuable insights, emotional support, and practical guidance to navigate your healthcare journey more effectively.

7.4 Online Health Information: Reliability and Safety

The internet has become a valuable source of health information, offering access to a wealth of medical resources. However, it is essential to be cautious and discerning when using online health information, as only some sources are reliable and accurate. Here is an overview of how to evaluate the reliability and safety of online health information:

7.4.1 Importance of Reliable Information

Health Decisions: Accurate health information is essential for making informed decisions about your well-being, medical conditions, and treatments.

Safety: Misleading or incorrect information can lead to ineffective or harmful health practices.

7.4.2 Evaluating Online Health Information

Source Credibility: Look for information from reputable sources such as government health agencies (e.g., CDC, WHO), medical organizations (e.g., American Heart Association), and academic institutions.

Authorship: Check if the information is written or reviewed by qualified healthcare professionals, medical experts, or researchers.

Date of Publication: Ensure the information is current and up-to-date, as medical knowledge and guidelines may change over time.

Bias and Objectivity: Evaluate whether the information is presented objectively and free from commercial or promotional interests.

7.4.3 Red Flags for Unreliable Information

Sensational Claims: Be cautious of websites or articles that make dramatic or unrealistic claims about treatments or cures.

Lack of Citations: Reliable sources should reference scientific studies or reputable medical literature.

Personal Anecdotes: Avoid relying solely on personal stories or anecdotes as evidence for medical information.

7.4.4 Verifying Medical Information

Confirm information from multiple reliable sources to ensure accuracy.

Consult your healthcare provider to verify the information and get personalized advice if in doubt.

7.4.5 Online Health Communities

Forums and Social Media: Participate in online health communities cautiously. While they can offer support, they may also present misinformation.

Expert Moderation: Look for communities with expert moderation to ensure that discussions are accurate and safe.

7.4.6 Official Health Websites

Government Agencies: Websites of government health agencies, such as the CDC and WHO, provide trustworthy information.

Medical Associations: Sites of reputable medical associations often offer accurate and updated information.

7.4.7 Telehealth and Virtual Visits

Telehealth services offer access to qualified healthcare providers who can provide accurate medical information and advice.

7.4.8 Health Literacy

Enhance your health literacy by critically evaluating health information and discerning reliable sources.

Navigating online health information requires careful consideration to ensure you are accessing accurate and safe knowledge. By following these guidelines and seeking information from reputable sources, you can make informed decisions about your health and well-being. Remember that your healthcare provider is an invaluable resource for addressing specific health concerns and receiving personalized medical advice.

8. Emergency Preparedness and First Aid

8.1 Basic First Aid Techniques

Basic first aid techniques are essential life skills that can make a significant difference in providing immediate assistance during emergencies. Preparing to offer first aid can help stabilize a person's condition and save lives before professional medical help arrives. Here is an overview of basic first-aid techniques:

8.1.1 Assessing the Situation

Before providing first aid, assess the scene for potential dangers to yourself and others. Make sure it is safe to approach the injured person.

Call emergency services (108 or local emergency number) for professional assistance if the situation is serious.

8.1.2 CPR (Cardiopulmonary Resuscitation)

CPR is a life-saving technique used when a person's heart has stopped beating. It involves chest compressions and rescue breaths.

If you need to be trained in CPR, you can perform hands-only CPR by providing chest compressions at a rate of about 100-120 compressions per minute.

If trained, combine chest compressions with rescue breaths (30 compressions followed by two breaths).

8.1.3 Choking

Heimlich Maneuver: For conscious adults and children, perform the Heimlich maneuver by delivering abdominal thrusts to dislodge a blockage in the airway.

Back Blows and Chest Thrusts: For infants and unconscious victims, use back blows and chest thrusts to clear the airway.

8.1.4 Bleeding and Wound Care

Apply direct pressure with a clean cloth or bandage to control wound bleeding.

Elevate the injured area above the heart to help reduce blood flow.

Apply pressure to specific pressure points to help control bleeding.

8.1.5 Burns

Run cool water over a burn for 10-20 minutes to help alleviate pain and prevent further damage.

Cover the burn with a clean, non-stick bandage or cloth to protect it.

8.1.6 Fractures and Sprains

Immobilize a fractured or injured limb by splinting it to prevent further movement.

Elevate the injured area to help reduce swelling.

8.1.7 Seizures

During a seizure, ensure the person's safety by gently guiding them away from hazards.

Place a soft object (such as a folded jacket) under the head to prevent injury.

8.1.8 Allergic Reactions

If the person has a severe allergic reaction and has an epinephrine auto-injector, administer it according to instructions.

8.1.9 Bites and Stings

Clean the area of the bite or sting with soap and water.

Use a blunt object to scrape away stingers from bee or wasp stings gently.

Remember that these basic first aid techniques are meant to provide immediate assistance until professional medical help arrives. It is essential to seek professional medical care for serious injuries or conditions. Consider taking a formal first aid and CPR course to learn these techniques in more detail and practice them under the guidance of trained instructors.

8.2 Creating a Personal Emergency Plan

Creating a personal emergency plan is essential to ensure the safety and well-being of you and your loved ones during various types of emergencies, such as natural disasters, medical crises, or other unforeseen events. A well-thought-out plan can help you respond effectively and make informed decisions when faced with unexpected situations. Here is a step-by-step guide to creating a personal emergency plan.

8.2.1 Assess Potential Risks

Identify Hazards: Consider the types of disasters or emergencies likely to occur in your area, such as earthquakes, hurricanes, floods, or power outages.

Assess Vulnerabilities: Determine how these hazards might affect your home, family members, and daily routines.

8.2.2 Develop Your Plan

Establish a reliable communication plan to stay in touch with family members and friends during emergencies. Determine a designated meeting place and an out-of-area contact person.

Create a list of important contacts, including local emergency services, medical professionals, neighbors, and relatives.

Compile medical information for each family member, including allergies, medications, and medical conditions. Keep this information in a readily accessible location.

If evacuation is necessary, identify multiple routes from your home and a safe temporary location, such as a friend's house or a shelter.

Include pets in your emergency plan if you have pets. Identify pet-friendly shelters or accommodations.

Assemble an emergency kit that includes essentials such as water, non-perishable food, medications, a flashlight, batteries, a first aid kit, and essential documents.

Keep some cash on hand, as ATMs and credit card machines may not be accessible during emergencies.

Secure heavy furniture, appliances, and objects that could become hazards during earthquakes or storms.

Learn how to safely turn off gas, water, and electricity in emergencies.

8.2.3 Practice and Review

Family Drills: Regularly practice emergency scenarios with your family, including evacuation procedures, meeting points, and communication.

Kit Maintenance: Check and update your emergency kit periodically to ensure that food, water, and supplies remain usable.

Information Updates: Keep your emergency contacts and medical information up to date.

8.2.4 Stay Informed

Sign up for local emergency alerts and government agencies or community organizations notifications.

Stay informed about weather conditions and forecasts that could lead to emergencies.

8.2.5 Tailor Your Plan

Specific Needs: Consider the unique needs of family members, such as infants, elderly individuals, or those with disabilities.

Cultural or Religious Considerations: Incorporate any cultural or religious practices that might affect your emergency response.

Creating a personal emergency plan empowers you to take proactive steps to ensure the safety and well-being of yourself and your loved ones during unexpected events. Regularly review and update your plan to account for changes in circumstances and to ensure that everyone in your household is prepared and informed.

8.3 Recognizing Signs of Medical Emergencies

Recognizing signs of medical emergencies is crucial for taking prompt and appropriate action to provide assistance or seek professional medical help. Identifying the early warning signs of a medical crisis can significantly improve outcomes and potentially save lives. Here are some common signs of medical emergencies and how to respond:

8.3.1 Heart Attack

Chest pain or discomfort, pain radiating to the arm, jaw, or back, shortness of breath, sweating, nausea, light-headedness.

Call emergency services (108 or local emergency number) immediately. Keep the person calm, encourage them to sit and rest, and offer aspirin if available and not allergic.

8.3.2 Stroke

Sudden numbness or weakness in the face, arm, or leg (especially on one side of the body), confusion, trouble speaking or understanding, trouble seeing, and severe headache.

Act quickly by calling emergency services. Note when symptoms started, as it is essential information for medical treatment.

8.3.3 Severe Allergic Reaction (Anaphylaxis)

Difficulty breathing, swelling of the face, lips, or throat, hives, rapid heartbeat, nausea, confusion, and dizziness.

Administer an epinephrine auto-injector if available. Call emergency services and seek medical attention immediately.

8.3.4 Choking

Inability to speak or breathe, clutching the throat, making choking gestures.

If the person cannot cough, speak, or breathe, perform the Heimlich maneuver, back blows, and chest thrusts if they are unconscious or an infant.

8.3.5 Unconsciousness or Fainting

Sudden loss of consciousness, confusion, and inability to respond.

Ensure the person is lying on their back on a flat surface. Check for breathing and a pulse. If absent, begin CPR.

8.3.6 Seizures

Muscle twitching, jerking movements, loss of consciousness.

Protect the person from injury by moving dangerous objects away. Do not restrain them. Once the seizure stops, please place them safely and stay with them.

8.3.7 Difficulty Breathing

Rapid or labored breathing, wheezing, gasping for air.

Assist the person in a comfortable sitting position. If they have a prescribed inhaler, help them use it. Call for medical help if symptoms persist.

8.3.8 Bleeding

Profuse bleeding from a wound, bleeding that does not stop, rapid blood loss.

Apply direct pressure to the wound with a clean cloth or bandage. Elevate the injured area if possible. Seek medical help for severe bleeding.

8.3.9 Poisoning

Nausea, vomiting, confusion, dizziness, trouble breathing, changes in skin color, unusual odors.

Call poison control or emergency services. Provide as much information as possible about the substance ingested.

Recognizing these signs of medical emergencies and taking swift and appropriate action can help ensure the best possible outcome for needy individuals. Always call for professional medical help when in doubt or facing severe symptoms. Additionally, being trained in first aid and CPR can enhance your ability to respond effectively in medical emergencies.

9. Appendix

9.1 Case Studies

Case Study 1: Cardiovascular Health Counseling

Scenario: You are a pharmacist counseling a middle-aged patient recently diagnosed with hypertension. The patient is hesitant about starting medication due to concerns about side effects. How would you approach this counseling session and address the patient's concerns?

Case Study 2: Diabetes Management Education

Scenario: As a nurse, you are educating a newly diagnosed diabetic patient on insulin administration and self-monitoring of blood glucose levels. The patient is anxious and unsure about the process. Develop a step-by-step counseling plan to guide the patient through the education session.

Case Study 3: Smoking Cessation Support

Scenario: You are a physician counseling a long-term smoker who is ready to quit. The patient has attempted quitting before but relapsed. How do you tailor your counseling approach to enhance the patient's motivation and increase their chances of successfully quitting this time?

Case Study 4: Pediatric Asthma Care

Scenario: You are a pediatrician counseling parents of a child with asthma. The parents are having trouble understanding how to use an inhaler with a spacer device for their young child. Create a counseling session plan that addresses their concerns and provides clear instructions.

Case Study 5: Geriatric Polypharmacy Management

Scenario: As a geriatric pharmacist, you are reviewing the medication regimen of an elderly patient who is taking multiple medications from different healthcare providers. The patient is experiencing side effects and confusion. Develop a counseling approach to streamline the medication regimen and ensure patient safety.

Case Study 6: Mental Health Support

Scenario: You are a mental health counselor providing therapy to a young adult experiencing anxiety and depression. The patient is resistant to medication and prefers non-pharmacological approaches. Design a counseling session incorporating evidence-based techniques to address the patient's mental health needs.

For each case study, describe the scenario briefly, the challenges or issues involved, and a step-by-step outline of how a healthcare professional can approach the counseling session. Include key communication techniques, patient-centered strategies, and relevant resources from your handbook that the reader can refer to while working through the case study.

Interactive case studies encourage readers to think critically, apply theoretical knowledge to practical situations, and develop problem-solving skills. They can effectively reinforce the concepts presented in your patient counseling handbook and help readers become more confident and competent in real-world patient interactions.

9.2 Real-Life Patient Scenarios and Counseling Approaches

Absolutely, real-life patient scenarios and counseling approaches can be incredibly valuable. They provide practical examples of how healthcare professionals can apply their knowledge and skills in different situations. Here are a few sample patient scenarios and counseling approaches that you could include:

Scenario 1: Cardiovascular Health Counseling

Patient: John, a 55-year-old man with hypertension and high cholesterol.

Counseling Approach: Discuss the importance of medication adherence, lifestyle modifications (diet and exercise), and regular blood pressure and cholesterol monitoring. Provide resources for heart-healthy recipes and exercise plans.

Scenario 2: Diabetes Management Education

Patient: Sarah, a 30-year-old woman newly diagnosed with type 2 diabetes.

Counseling Approach: Teach Sarah about blood glucose monitoring, insulin administration, meal planning, and the impact of lifestyle choices on diabetes management. Emphasize the significance of balanced nutrition and physical activity.

Scenario 3: Smoking Cessation Support

Patient: Michael, a 40-year-old smoker who wants to quit.

Counseling Approach: Employ motivational interviewing techniques to explore Michael's reasons for quitting. Offer nicotine replacement options, create a quit plan with coping strategies, and schedule follow-up sessions for ongoing support.

Scenario 4: Pediatric Asthma Care

Patient: Emily, a 7-year-old girl with newly diagnosed asthma.

Counseling Approach: Educate Emily's parents about asthma triggers, proper inhaler technique with a spacer, and the importance of an asthma action plan. Provide resources for recognizing early signs of an asthma attack.

Scenario 5: Geriatric Polypharmacy Management

Patient: Mr. Anderson, an 80-year-old man taking multiple medications.

Counseling Approach: Conduct a comprehensive medication review, assess potential drug interactions, and simplify the medication regimen. Discuss the importance of medication adherence and encourage open communication with all healthcare providers.

Scenario 6: Mental Health Support

Patient: Maria, a 25-year-old with anxiety and depression.

Counseling Approach: Use active listening and empathy to understand Maria's feelings. Discuss the benefits of therapy, medication options, and stress reduction techniques. Develop a personalized wellness plan and encourage regular check-ins.

Scenario 7: Women's Health and Reproductive Counseling

Patient: Lisa, a 30-year-old woman seeking contraception options.

Counseling Approach: Present a range of contraceptive methods, discuss their effectiveness, potential side effects, and address Lisa's preferences and concerns. Provide information about regular check-ups and screenings.

Scenario 8: Chronic Pain Management

Patient: James, a 60-year-old man with chronic back pain.

Counseling Approach: Explore James' pain history, lifestyle factors, and previous treatments. Discuss non-pharmacological pain management strategies (exercise, physical therapy) alongside medication options, emphasizing the importance of a balanced approach.

For each scenario, outline the patient's background, concerns, and health goals. Then, provide a step-by-step counseling approach, highlighting communication techniques, empathy, and evidence-based practices that healthcare professionals can use to guide their interactions. Including both successful and challenging scenarios can help prepare readers for various real-world counseling situations.

9.3 Brief on Different types of Patient Counselling Forms

Including sample patient counseling forms in your patient counseling handbook can provide healthcare professionals with practical tools they can use in their practice. Here are a few examples of patient counseling forms that you could include:

Medication Counseling Checklist

Healthcare professionals can use this form to ensure that they cover all essential information when counseling a patient about a new medication. It could include sections for dosage instructions, potential side effects, drug interactions, and any special instructions.

Treatment Plan Worksheet

A treatment plan worksheet can help healthcare professionals collaborate with patients to develop a personalized treatment plan. It could include spaces to outline treatment goals, medications, lifestyle changes, and follow-up appointments.

Inhaler Technique Assessment Form

This form could be used for patients using inhalers to assess and document their inhaler technique during counseling sessions. It could include a checklist of proper steps for inhaler use and areas for notes on improvements or adjustments needed.

Diabetes Self-Management Log:

A diabetes self-management log can help patients track their blood sugar levels, medication doses, dietary choices, and physical activity. This form can facilitate patient self-monitoring and provide healthcare professionals with valuable insights during counseling sessions.

Tobacco Cessation Progress Tracker:

For patients trying to quit smoking, a progress tracker can help them record their quit attempts, triggers, coping strategies, and cravings. This form can assist healthcare professionals in tailoring counseling sessions to the patient's specific needs.

Mental Health Wellness Plan:

For patients managing mental health conditions, a wellness plan can outline strategies for self-care, stress management, and coping techniques. It could include spaces for patients to set goals and track their emotional well-being over time.

Pediatric Immunization Schedule

A pediatric immunization schedule can help parents of young children keep track of their child's vaccination appointments and upcoming immunizations. This form can serve as a visual reminder and facilitate discussions about vaccine schedules.

Chronic Disease Management Diary

Patients with chronic conditions could use a management diary to track symptoms, medication adherence, and lifestyle factors. Healthcare professionals can review the diary during counseling sessions to identify trends and make informed adjustments to the treatment plan.

Nutritional Intake Journal

A nutritional intake journal can assist patients in tracking their daily food and fluid intake. This form can be helpful for dietitians and nutritionists during counseling sessions to provide personalized dietary recommendations.

Follow-Up Appointment Reminder Card

A simple reminder card that patients can take home can help them remember their upcoming follow-up appointments. This can enhance continuity of care and ensure that patients receive necessary follow-up counseling.

Remember, each form should be designed with clarity and simplicity, making it easy for healthcare professionals and patients to use. Provide clear instructions on filling out the form and suggest how it can be incorporated into patient interactions. You can also create these forms digitally for easy printing or electronic sharing.

9.4 Glossary of Medical Terms

Here is a glossary of medical terms to help you understand key concepts and terminology related to healthcare and medicine:

Anatomy: The study of the structure and organization of the body.

Biopsy: The removal and examination of a small tissue sample from the body to diagnose or monitor a medical condition.

Cardiovascular: About the heart and blood vessels.

Diagnosis: Identifying a disease or medical condition based on signs, symptoms, and diagnostic tests.

Endocrine System: The system of glands that secrete hormones to regulate bodily functions and processes.

Fracture: A break or crack in a bone.

Gastrointestinal: Relating to the stomach and intestines, also known as the digestive system.

Hematology: The study of blood and blood disorders.

Immunization: Introducing a vaccine stimulates the immune system and provides immunity against a specific disease.

Jaundice: Yellowing of the skin and eyes, often indicative of liver or bile duct problems.

Kidney: A pair of organs that filter waste products from the blood and produce urine.

Lung: One of the two organs responsible for respiration and gas exchange in the body.

Metabolism: The chemical processes that occur within a living organism to maintain life.

Neurology: The branch of medicine deals with the nervous system and its disorders.

Oncology: The study and treatment of cancer.

Pediatrics: The branch of medicine that focuses on children's health and medical care.

Quality of Life: An individual's overall well-being and satisfaction, including physical, emotional, and social aspects.

Radiology: The branch of medicine that uses imaging techniques such as X-rays, CT scans, and MRI to diagnose and treat diseases.

Surgery: The medical specialty involves operative procedures to treat diseases, injuries, or conditions.

Therapy: Medical treatment designed to alleviate symptoms or improve a person's health.

Ultrasound: An imaging technique that uses high-frequency sound waves to produce images of the inside of the body.

Vaccination: The administration of a vaccine to stimulate the immune system and provide protection against specific diseases.

Wound: An injury to the body that breaks the skin or internal tissues.

Aneurysm: An abnormal bulging or ballooning of a blood vessel, often caused by weakness in the vessel walls.

Arrhythmia: Irregular or abnormal heart rhythms that can affect the heart's ability to pump blood effectively.

Aspiration is inhaling foreign substances, such as food or liquid, into the airways or lungs.

Biopsy: The removal and examination of a small tissue sample from the body to diagnose or monitor a medical condition.

Catheter: A thin, flexible tube inserted into the body to administer fluids, drain fluids, or perform medical procedures.

Contraindication: A factor or condition that makes a specific treatment or medication potentially harmful or inappropriate.

Dementia: A group of cognitive disorders characterized by memory loss, impaired thinking, and personality changes.

Electrocardiogram (ECG or EKG): A test that records the heart's electrical activity to evaluate its rhythm and function.

Endoscopy: A flexible tube with a camera is used to examine the inside of organs or body cavities.

Fever: Elevated body temperature is often caused by infections or inflammatory processes.

Gastroenteritis: Inflammation of the stomach and intestines, commonly known as stomach flu.

Hematology: The branch of medicine that deals with blood and blood disorders.

Intravenous (IV): About administering fluids, medications, or nutrients directly into a vein.

Jaundice: Yellowing of the skin and eyes due to elevated bilirubin levels in the blood.

Lymph Nodes: Small, bean-shaped structures that filter lymph and play a role in immune responses.

Migraine: A severe headache often accompanied by visual disturbances, nausea, and sensitivity to light and sound.

Nephrology: The medical specialty focuses on the kidneys and their functions.

Ophthalmology: The branch of medicine that deals with the eyes and vision.

Pneumonia: Inflammation of the lungs caused by infection, leading to symptoms such as cough, fever, and difficulty breathing.

Quarantine: Isolation of individuals exposed to infectious diseases to prevent their spread.

Radiation: High-energy particles or waves used in medical imaging, cancer treatment, and other applications.

Stethoscope: A medical instrument used to listen to internal sounds of the body, such as heart and lung sounds.

Thrombosis: The formation of a blood clot within a blood vessel can lead to severe complications.

Urology: The medical specialty focused on the urinary system and male reproductive organs.

Vital Signs: Essential physiological measurements, including heart rate, blood pressure, respiratory rate, and body temperature.

X-ray: A medical imaging technique that uses electromagnetic radiation to create images of internal structures.

Zoonosis: A disease that can be transmitted from animals to humans.

Medical terminology is vast and diverse, and these additional terms provide a glimpse into the complex world of healthcare and medicine. Medical definitions can vary based on context and medical specialties, so it is important to consult medical professionals and trusted resources for accurate information.

References

Books:

1. "Motivational Interviewing: Helping People Change" by William R. Miller and Stephen Rollnick

2. "Communication Skills for Pharmacists: Building Relationships, Improving Patient Care" by Bruce A. Berger

3. "Clinical Guidelines for Assessment and Management of Chronic Pain" by Institute of Medicine

4. "The Diabetes Textbook: Clinical Principles, Patient Management, and Public Health Issues" edited by Joel Rodriguez-Saldana

5. "Counseling Patients About Sexual Health and Reproductive Issues" by Judith A. Lewis and Michael D. Hager

Clinical Guidelines and Resources:

6. Centers for Disease Control and Prevention (CDC) - Guidelines for Various Medical Conditions

7. American Heart Association (AHA) - Guidelines for Cardiovascular Health

8. American Diabetes Association (ADA) - Standards of Medical Care in Diabetes

9. National Institute on Drug Abuse (NIDA) - Resources for Substance Abuse Counseling

10. American Psychological Association (APA) - Resources for Mental Health Counseling

Patient Counseling Handbook

Journals and Articles:

11. The New England Journal of Medicine

12. Journal of the American Medical Association (JAMA)

13. Journal of Clinical Pharmacy and Therapeutics

14. Patient Education and Counseling

15. Journal of Diabetes Science and Technology

Websites and Online Resources:

16. Mayo Clinic Patient Care and Health Information

17. WebMD - Trusted Health and Medical Information

18. National Institutes of Health (NIH) - Health Information

19. MedlinePlus - Health Topics and Medication Information

20. RxList - Comprehensive Medication Information

Professional Organizations:

21. American Pharmacists Association (APhA)

22. American Nurses Association (ANA)

23. American Psychological Association (APA)

24. American Academy of Family Physicians (AAFP)

25. American College of Physicians (ACP)

Government Agencies:

26. U.S. Food and Drug Administration (FDA)

27. National Institute of Mental Health (NIMH)

28. National Heart, Lung, and Blood Institute (NHLBI)

29. National Institute on Aging (NIA)

www.ingramcontent.com/pod-product-compliance
Lightning Source LLC
Chambersburg PA
CBHW072220170526
45158CB00002BA/674